Veterinary Emergency and Critical Care Procedures

Second Edition

Veterinary Emergency and Critical Care Procedures

Second Edition

Timothy B. Hackett
Elisa M. Mazzaferro

WILEY Blackwell

This edition first published 2012 © 2012 by John Wiley & Sons, Inc
First edition published 2006 © Blackwell Publishing

Wiley-Blackwell is an imprint of John Wiley & Sons, formed by the merger of Wiley's global Scientific, Technical and Medical business with Blackwell Publishing.

Editorial Offices
2121 State Avenue, Ames, Iowa 50014-8300, USA
The Atrium, Southern Gate, Chichester, West Sussex, PO19 8SQ, UK
9600 Garsington Road, Oxford, OX4 2DQ, UK

For details of our global editorial offices, for customer services and for information about how to apply for permission to reuse the copyright material in this book please see our website at www.wiley.com/wiley-blackwell.

Library of Congress Cataloging-in-Publication Data

Hackett, Tim B.
Veterinary emergency and critical care procedures / Timothy B. Hackett, Elisa M. Mazzaferro.
2nd ed.
    p.   cm.
   Includes bibliographical references and index.
   ISBN 978-0-470-95855-1 (pbk. : alk. paper)
1. Veterinary emergencies.   2. Veterinary critical care.   I. Mazzaferro, Elisa M.   II. Title.
SF778.H33 2012
636.089′6025–dc23

2012007649

A catalogue record for this book is available from the British Library.

Wiley also publishes its books in a variety of electronic formats. Some content that appears in print may not be available in electronic books.

Set in 10/12pt Times by SPi Publisher Services, Pondicherry, India

Disclaimer

SKY10081374_081224

Contents

Preface,   vii

1 Vascular Access Techniques,   1

2 Nutritional Support and Orogastric Lavage,   69

3 Thoracocentesis and Thoracostomy Tube Placement,   101

4 Oxygen Supplementation and Respiratory Sampling Techniques,   133

5 Urinary Catheter Placement, Urohydropulsion, and Temporary Antepubic
   Cystostomy Catheter Placement,   171

6 Abdominocentesis and Diagnostic Peritoneal Lavage,   209

7 Pericardiocentesis and Pericardial Drainage Catheter,   233

8 Central Venous Pressure,   243

9 Cardiopulmonary Resuscitation,   253

10 Continuous Rate Infusions,   273

Index,   277

The companion website provides video clips demonstrating procedures
from the book for download at

www.wiley.com/go/hackett

Preface

The first edition of this text came about when we realized that there were no textbooks with clear step-by-step photos of emergency procedures that can be used to save lives. While these procedures may be intuitive for an emergency clinician, they are often performed infrequently by those who are fortunate to work in busy day practices and whose patients are often healthy and need wellness care. Thus, the concept for the original text was born. The text is divided into sections, each with a series of procedures that are organized to walk the clinician step by step through the procedures from start to finish. Each photo has a caption for clarification of instructions, and some have helpful hints to avoid complications or frustration.

The photos in this edition are in color, which is a great and added benefit from the authors' perspective. The most exciting addition to this edition is a video counterpart to many of the procedures, which will help with teaching and refreshing the clinician's memory. This material is meant to be a useful teaching tool for veterinarians, veterinary technicians, and students to improve clinical skills and knowledge, and to help save the lives of veterinary patients.

TBH, EMM

CHAPTER 1

Vascular Access Techniques

INTRODUCTION

A variety of methods can be used for placement of peripheral, central venous, and arterial catheters. If a peripheral or central catheter cannot be placed due to small patient size, severe hypovolemia or dehydration, or hypotension, intraosseous catheters can be placed in the femur, humerus, or wing of the ileum. This chapter will discuss indications, contraindications, and methodologies listed above.

Through-the-needle catheters or over-the-wire central venous catheters can be placed in the jugular, medial saphenous, or lateral saphenous veins. The indications and contraindications for central venous catheter placement, irrespective of type, are similar.

CENTRAL VENOUS CATHETER PLACEMENT

Introduction

Central venous catheters can be placed into the jugular, lateral saphenous, and medial saphenous veins. Central venous catheters can be used for infusion of colloid and crystalloid fluids, infusion of continuous or intermittent drugs, and infusion of hyperosmolar solutions including parenteral nutrition. Catheters placed into the jugular vein can be used for measurement of central venous pressure to guide fluid therapy and help avoid volume overload. An additional benefit of indwelling central venous catheters is ease of repeated blood sample collection without the need for repeated venipuncture.

Supplies Needed

Antimicrobial scrub and solution
Central venous catheter(s)

Veterinary Emergency and Critical Care Procedures, Second Edition. Timothy B. Hackett and Elisa M. Mazzaferro.
© 2012 John Wiley & Sons, Inc. Published 2012 by John Wiley & Sons, Inc.

Cotton roll gauze
Electric clipper
Electric clipper blades
Gauze, 4-×4-inch squares
Heparinized flush
Kling or gauze bandaging material
T-port
1-inch white tape

Indications

Large volume crystalloid or colloid infusion
Continuous drug infusion
Repeated blood sample collection
Infusion of parenteral nutrition or other hyperosmolar substances
Central venous pressure measurement

Contraindications

Coagulopathies
   Thrombocytopenia
   Thrombocytopathia
   Vitamin K antagonist rodenticide
Hypercoagulable states
   Hyperadrenocorticism
   Disseminated intravascular coagulation (DIC)
   Protein losing enteropathy
   Protein losing nephropathy
Catheters should not be placed in the jugular vein in cases of increased intraocular or
      intracranial pressure or thrombosis of one jugular vein

 Video available online

Go to www.wiley.com/go/hackett to view a video of this procedure.

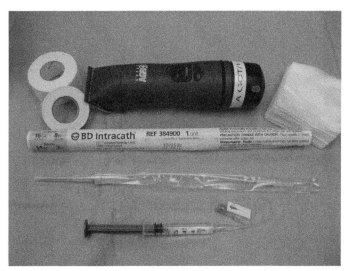

Fig. 1.1. Set-up for central venous through-the-needle catheter placement.

Helpful hint: Have all components ready before restraining the patient and attempting to place the catheter.

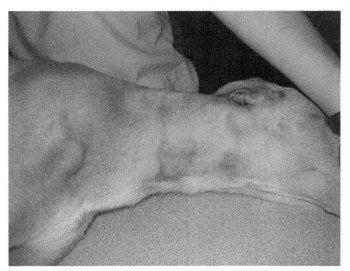

Fig. 1.2. Place the patient in lateral recumbency. Clip the jugular furrow from the ramus of the mandible caudally to the thoracic inlet and dorsally and ventrally to midline.

Helpful hint: In long-haired patients, make sure to clip the "feathers" that might lay over your field.

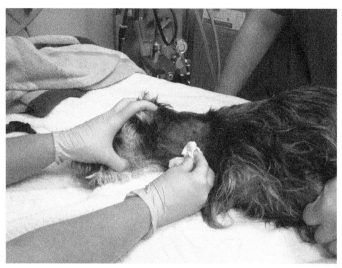

Fig. 1.3. Aseptically scrub the clipped area.

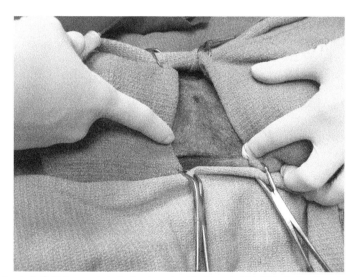

Fig. 1.4. Drape the sterile field, then occlude the jugular vein at the thoracic inlet. Note the jugular vein under the skin.

Helpful hint: In overweight patients, the jugular vein may not be visible, even after occlusion at the thoracic inlet.

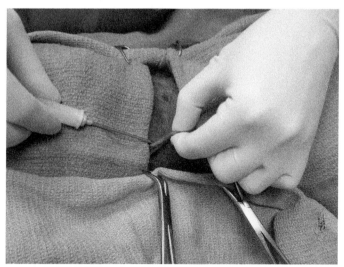

Fig. 1.5. Wearing sterile gloves, tent the skin over the proposed site of catheter insertion, and insert the needle through the skin.

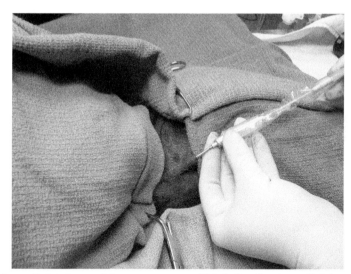

Fig. 1.6. Insert the needle into the vessel. In some cases, you will feel a "pop" as the needle is inserted into the vessel. Watch for a flash of blood in the catheter. Once a flash of blood is observed, push the catheter through the needle into the vein.

Helpful hint: In extremely hypotensive or hypovolemic patients, a flash of blood may not occur.

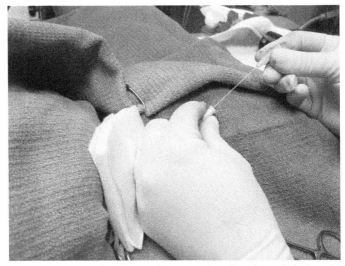

Fig. 1.7. Once the catheter is pushed to the hub securely, remove the stylette from within the catheter.

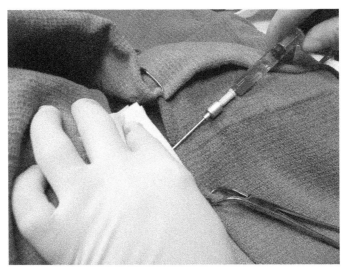

Fig. 1.8. Flush the catheter with heparinized saline.

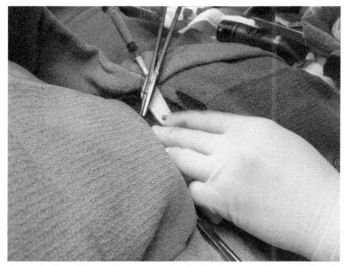

Fig. 1.9. Remove the needle from the vessel, and secure the plastic pieces over the needle for safety.

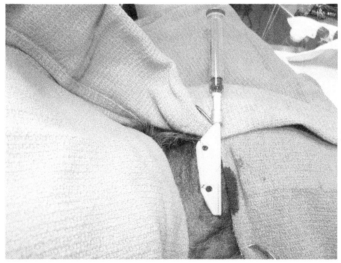

Fig. 1.10. Suture the plastic pieces and catheter hub in place to the skin.

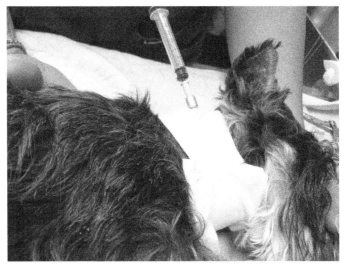

Fig. 1.11. Place sterile gauze squares over the site of catheter insertion, and bandage in place first with lengths of 1-inch adhesive tape.

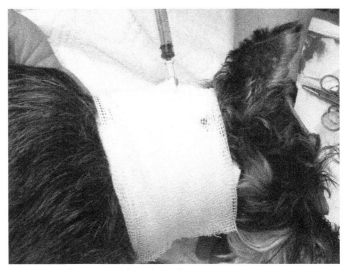

Fig. 1.12. Next, secure cotton roll gauze over the catheter site.

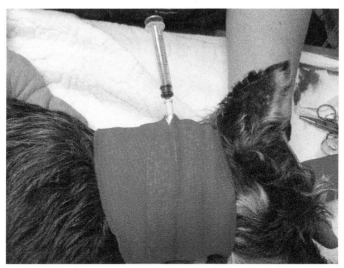

Fig. 1.13. Finally, secure a final outer layer over the catheter bandage.

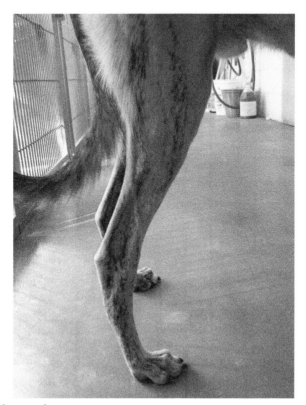

Fig. 1.14. Lateral saphenous vein.

(a)

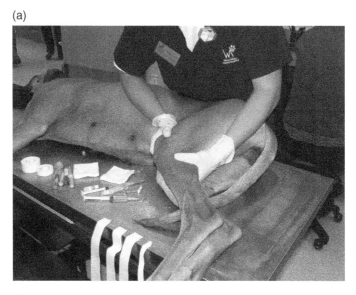

(b)

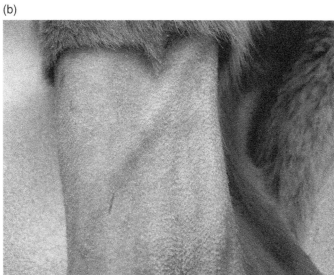

Fig. 1.15. Place the patient in lateral recumbency (Fig. 1.15a) and have an assistant restrain. Clip the distal limb circumferentially in between the stifle and hock, over the lateral saphenous vein. Have an assistant occlude the vessel proximally, and visualize the vessel as it courses under the skin. Aseptically scrub with antimicrobial cleansing solution (Fig. 1.15b).

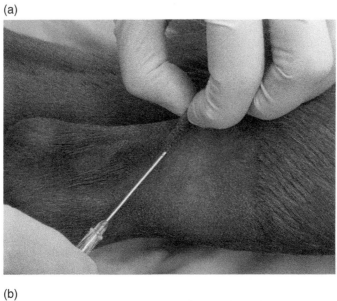

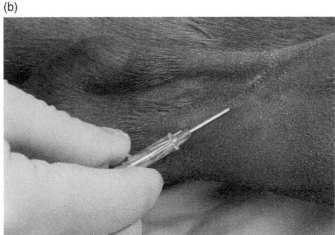

Fig. 1.16. Tent the skin over the vessel and insert the through-the-needle catheter through the skin (Fig. 1.16a), then into the vessel, bevel up (Fig. 1.16b). Watch for a flash of blood in the catheter.

Helpful hint: To hold the vessel in place while you are attempting to insert the catheter, pull the skin tightly around the back of the leg.

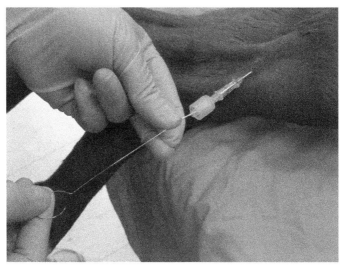

Fig. 1.17. Insert the catheter to the hub, then push the through-the-needle catheter and stylette into the vessel.

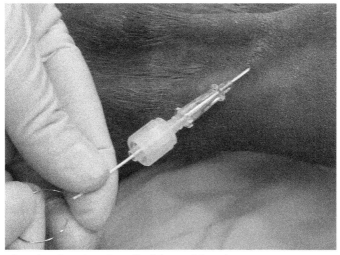

Fig. 1.18. Remove the stylette from the catheter. Don't let go of the catheter.

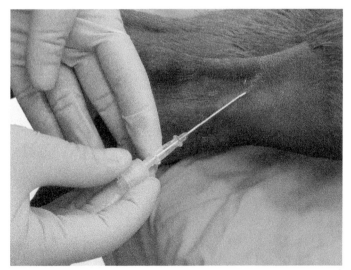

Fig. 1.19. Pull the needle and hub off of the catheter, leaving the catheter in the vessel. Don't let go of the catheter.

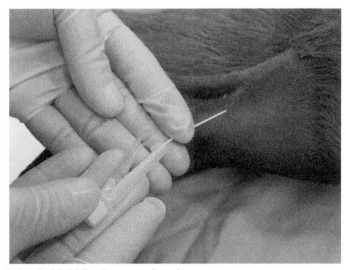

Fig. 1.20. Place the luer-lock hub/clip adapter over the catheter.

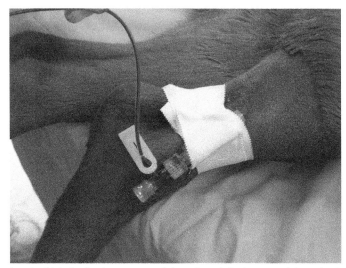

Fig. 1.21. Place a length of 1-inch adhesive tape around the catheter hub, then around the patient's limb. Next, flush the catheter with heparinized saline.

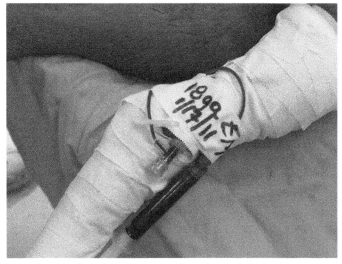

Fig. 1.22. Wrap a second length of tape under, then around the catheter. Next, wrap bandage material around the limb, then secure tape over the catheter and T-port. Label the catheter. It is now ready for use.

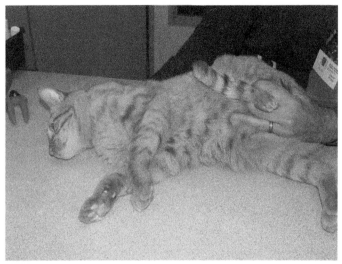

Fig. 1.23. Place the patient in lateral recumbancy and have an assistant restrain. Clip the rear limb circumferentially in between the stifle and hock.

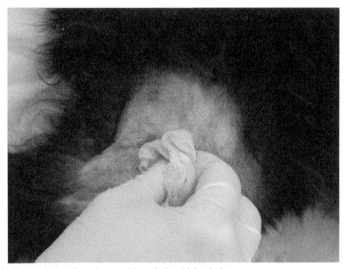

Fig. 1.24. Aseptically scrub the clipped area with antimicrobial solution.

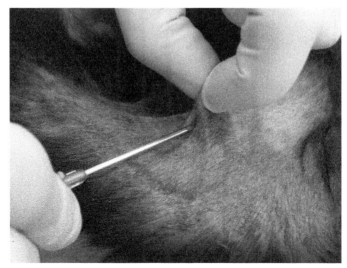

Fig. 1.25. Pull the skin tightly around the leg to keep the vein from rolling under the skin. Insert the needle through the skin just adjacent to the vessel. Avoid lacerating or puncturing the vessel.

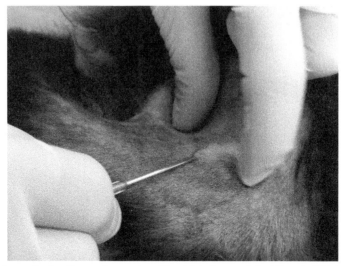

Fig. 1.26. Place the needle directly over the vessel, and insert into the vessel at a 15° angle. Watch for a flash of blood in the catheter. Insert the catheter into the vessel.

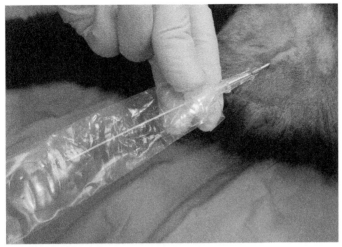

Fig. 1.27. Insert the catheter through the needle, into the vessel.

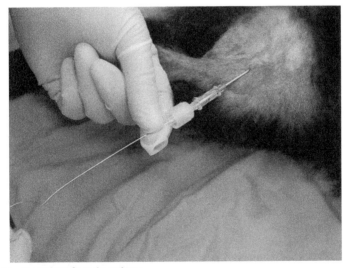

Fig. 1.28. Withdraw the stylette from the catheter.

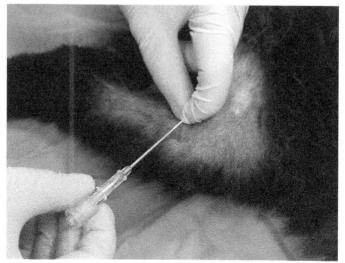

Fig. 1.29. Remove the needle off of the catheter. Take care to not let go of the catheter.

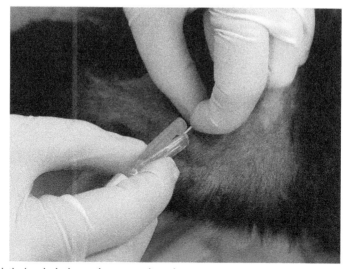

Fig. 1.30. Attach the luer-lock clamp adapter onto the catheter.

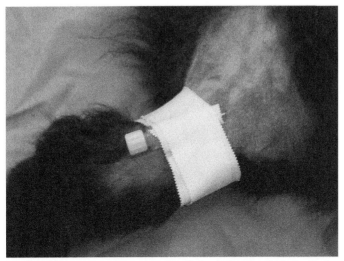

Fig. 1.31. Secure the catheter hub to the medial aspect of the limb with lengths of 1-inch adhesive tape.

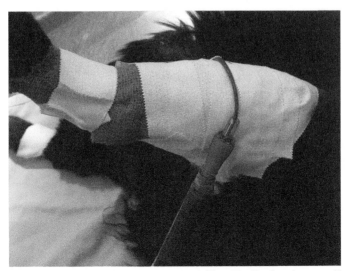

Fig. 1.32. Bandage the limb in layers of cotton roll gauze, Vetrap™, or Elastikon®, and secure a T-port that has been flushed with heparinized saline to the lateral aspect of the limb for easy access.

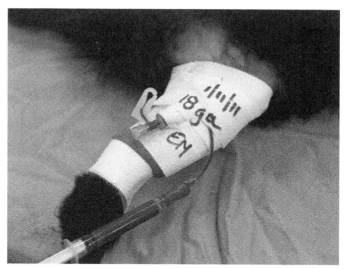

Fig. 1.33. Label the catheter bandage, and the catheter is ready for use.

OVER-THE-WIRE CATHETERS (SELDINGER TECHNIQUE)

Introduction

Over-the-wire (Seldinger) central venous catheters can be placed into the jugular, lateral saphenous, and medial saphenous veins. Central venous catheters can be used for infusion of colloid and crystalloid fluids, infusion of continuous or intermittent drugs, and infusion of hyperosmolar solutions including parenteral nutrition. Catheters placed into the jugular vein can be used for measurement of central venous pressure to guide fluid therapy and help avoid volume overload. An additional benefit of indwelling central venous catheters is ease of repeated blood sample collection without the need for repeated venipuncture. Many companies supply single- and multi-lumen over-the-wire products. Multi-lumen catheters are beneficial when multiple products are being infused into a patient simultaneously. The added ports allow vascular access without the need for placement of multiple single-lumen central or peripheral venous catheters.

Supplies Needed

Sterile gloves
Antimicrobial scrub solution
Number 11 scalpel blade
2% lidocaine
3-ml syringe with 24-gauge needle
Electric clipper and blades
1-inch white tape
3–0 nonabsorbable suture
Over-the-wire single or multi-lumen catheter kit
   Over-the-needle IV catheter
   Over-the-wire long catheter
   Vascular dilator
   Wire for catheter introduction into vessel
Needle holders
Suture scissors
Gauze, 4-×4-inch squares
Cotton bandage material
Kling
Elastikon® or Vetrap™

Indications

Frequent blood sample collection
Infusion of multiple drugs, fluids, blood products, or parenteral nutrition
Measurement of central venous pressure

Contraindications

Venous thrombosis
Coagulopathies
Should not be placed in jugular vein in cases of increased intracranial pressure

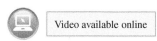 Video available online

Go to www.wiley.com/go/hackett to view a video of this procedure.

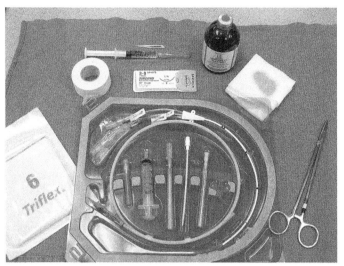

Fig. 1.34. Supplies needed for over-the-wire catheter.

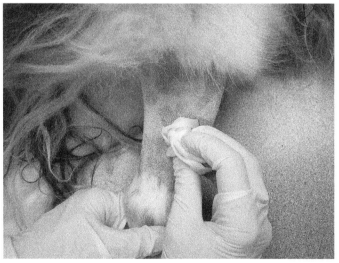

Fig. 1.35. Clip and aseptically scrub over the proposed site of catheter placement.

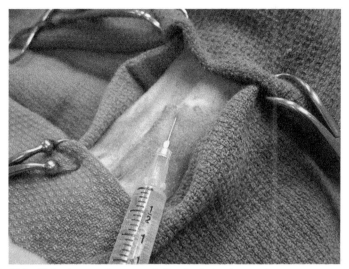

Fig. 1.36. Insert a bleb of lidocaine over the proposed site of catheter placement.

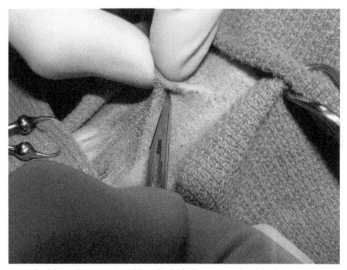

Fig. 1.37. Make a small incision with a number 11 scalpel blade through the skin. Make sure to not nick the underlying vessel.

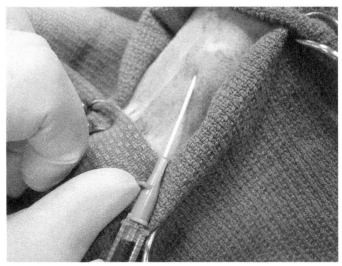

Fig. 1.38. Tent the skin and insert the over-the needle catheter through the skin, and direct the catheter and stylette into the vessel.

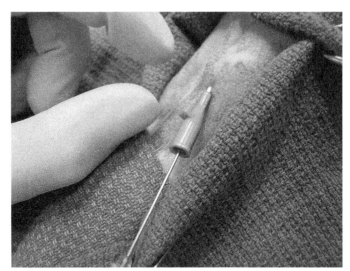

Fig. 1.39. Once the catheter is seated in the vessel, remove the stylette from the catheter. The catheter should bleed freely.

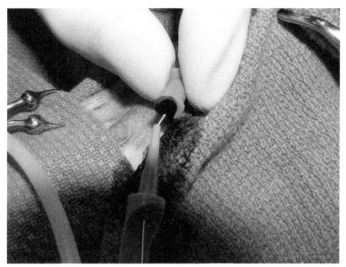

Fig. 1.40. Draw the "J" back into the introducer. Gently seat the introducer into the catheter hub, and insert the wire through the catheter hub into the vessel. Make sure to never let go of the wire.

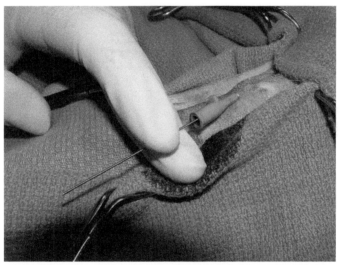

Fig. 1.41. Once the wire is inserted into the vessel, remove the catheter from the vessel, and over the wire. The wire alone will be left in the vessel.

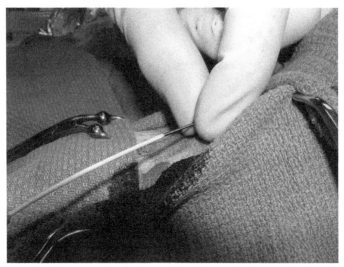

Fig. 1.42. Push the vascular dilator over the wire, through the skin, and into the vessel a short distance to enlarge the opening in the subcutaneous tissues and vessel.

Helpful hint: Hold the vascular dilator as near the skin as possible, and push with a twisting motion into the vessel.

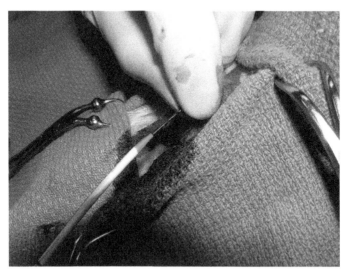

Fig. 1.43. Remove the vascular dilator from over the wire, and flush all ports of the over-the-wire catheter. Insert the catheter over the wire. Pull the wire slowly out of the vessel and feed it into the catheter. The wire will eventually appear out of one of the proximal ports of the catheter. Grasp the wire, and feed the catheter into the vessel.

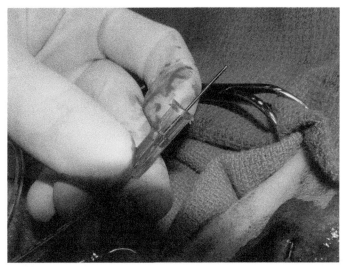

Fig. 1.44. The wire will eventually appear out of one of the proximal ports of the catheter. Grasp the wire, and feed the catheter into the vessel.

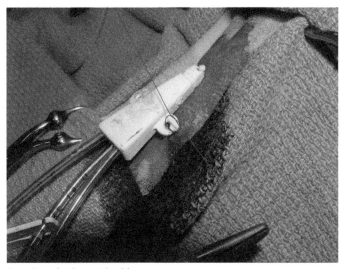

Fig. 1.45. Suture the catheter in place to the skin.

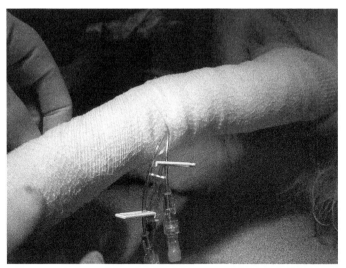

Fig. 1.46. Bandage the catheter, and label it.

Helpful hint: You have placed a large hole in the vessel. Remember to place a pressure bandage over this site when it comes time to remove the catheter, to prevent hemorrhage.

PERIPHERAL CATHETERIZATION

Introduction

Peripheral venous catheters are the most common type of intravenous catheter placed in small animal patients. Peripheral catheters are easy to place and simple to maintain, and have minimal risks to the patient. Peripheral catheters can be used for the infusion of crystalloid and colloid fluids, including blood products, and for the infusion of intravenous drugs and anesthetic agents. In large breeds, larger-bore (16- to 18-gauge) catheters can sometimes be used for blood sample collection.

Supplies Needed

1/2- and 1-inch white adhesive tape to secure and wrap catheter
Kling or brown gauze
Permanent marker to label catheter bandage
Cotton balls
4- × 4-inch gauze squares
T-port or male adapter
Heparinized flush solution in 3-ml syringe
    1,000 units of nonfractionated heparin/250 to 500 ml 0.9% saline; bags of unused heparinized saline should be discarded after 24 hours
Antimicrobial scrub product
Electric clippers
Electric clipper blades
Intravenous catheter

Indications

Infusion of crystalloid and colloid fluids
Infusion of blood products
Infusion of intravenous drugs
Blood sample collection
Induce and maintain general anesthesia

Contraindications

Burn, abrasion, or pyoderma over catheter site
Thrombosis of catheter and vein selected for catheterization
Infusion of hyperoncotic solutions (parenteral nutrition)

 Video available online

Go to www.wiley.com/go/hackett to view a video of this procedure.

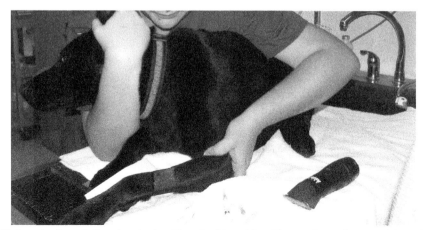

Fig. 1.47. Restraint for cephalic catheterization. The animal is positioned in sternal recumbency, and the assistant drapes one arm under the animal's neck, pulling the head toward the assistant's body, then pushes the forelimb cranially while occluding the vessel at the elbow.

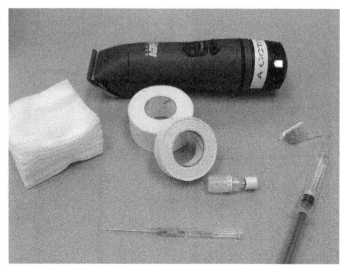

Fig. 1.48. Supplies needed for peripheral catheterization.

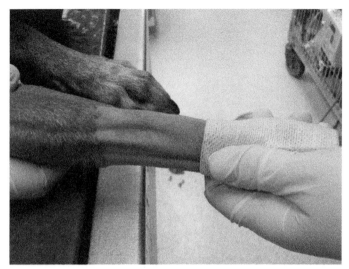

Fig. 1.49. Have an assistant restrain the patient and clip the antebrachium circumferentially in between the elbow and carpus, then aseptically scrub the clipped area.

Helpful hint: Remove any loose fur with a piece of dry 4-×4-inch gauze prior to scrubbing the limb.

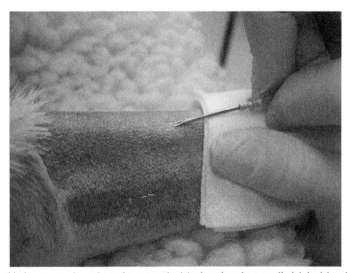

Fig. 1.50. If the skin is very tough, or the patient severely dehydrated, make a small nick incision through the skin with the bevel of an 18-gauge needle. This is called "percutaneous facilitation," and will make the task of catheter insertion easier.

Helpful hint: Use care to avoid lacerating the vessel during this procedure.

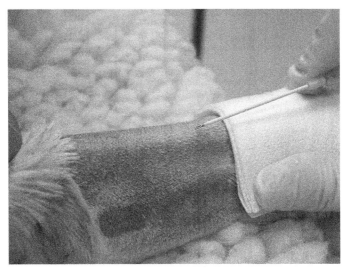

Fig. 1.51. Have an assistant occlude the vessel, then insert the needle through the skin at a 15° angle. Bluntly but gently penetrate the vein.

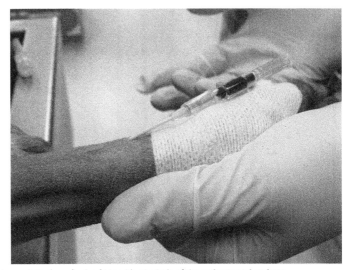

Fig. 1.52. Watch carefully for a flash of blood in the hub of the catheter and stylette.

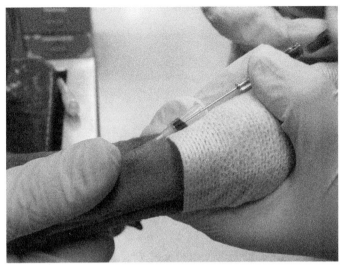

Fig. 1.53. Have an assistant occlude the vessel just over the point of catheter insertion, then remove the stylette.

Helpful hint: Having the assistant occlude the catheter during this step helps to prevent backflow of blood into your field.

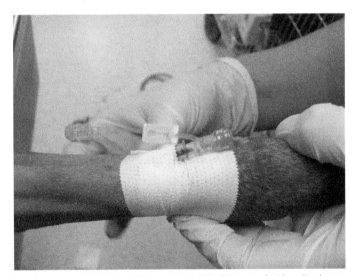

Fig. 1.54. Tape the catheter around the hub and limb with a half-inch length of white adhesive tape.

Helpful hint: Make sure that the catheter hub and skin are completely dry, so that the tape will securely attach itself to the catheter hub and the catheter will not spin around, or else the catheter will not remain in place and will pull out of the vessel.

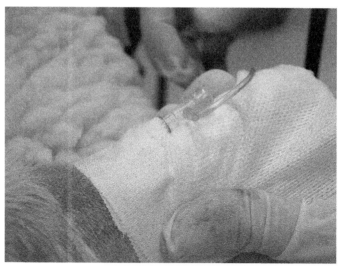

Fig. 1.55. Place a T-port flushed with heparinized saline and flush the catheter.

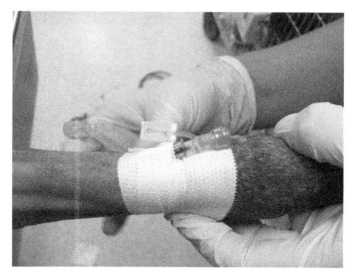

Fig. 1.56. Finish taping the catheter in place with layers of 1-inch white adhesive tape, Kling or brown gauze, Elastikon®, or Vetrap™.

Helpful hint: Label the top layer of tape with the size of the catheter, date of catheter placement, and initials of the person who placed the catheter.

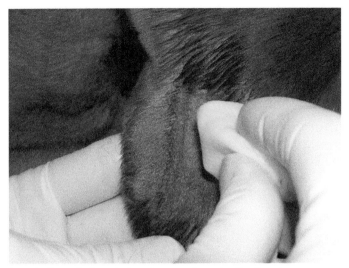

Fig. 1.57. Clip and aseptically scrub along the lateral ear margin to visualize the vein.

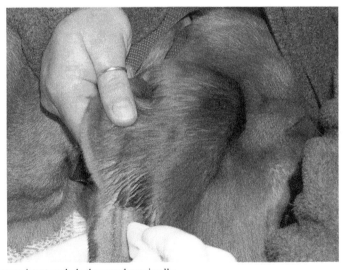

Fig. 1.58. Have an assistant occlude the vessel proximally.

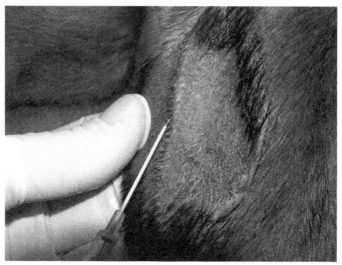

Fig. 1.59. Hold the ear in the non-dominant hand, and insert the over-the-needle catheter through the skin into the vessel. Watch for a flash of blood in the catheter hub.

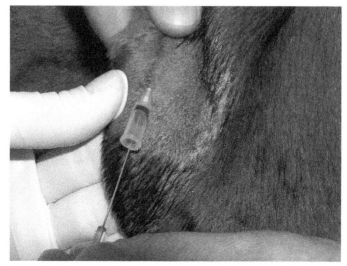

Fig. 1.60. Once a flash of blood is observed in the catheter hub, push the catheter off of the stylette, into the vessel.

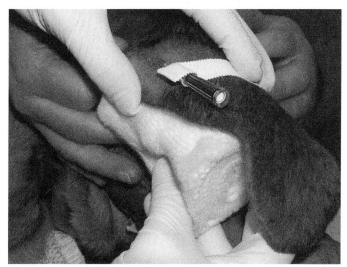

Fig. 1.61. Place a length of half-inch white tape around the catheter hub and around the ear. Place a roll of cotton gauze under the ear during catheter wrapping. The roll of cotton allows the ear to fold, rather than remain flat.

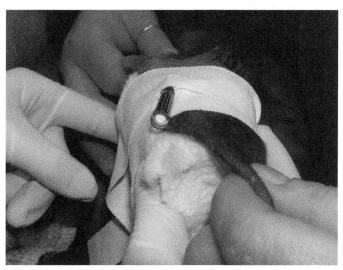

Fig. 1.62. Place a second length of 1-inch white tape under the catheter, and around the ear in a similar manner.

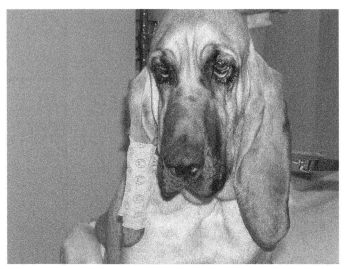
Fig. 1.63. Place nonadhesive bandage material over the catheter.

VASCULAR CUTDOWN

Introduction

In small animal patients with severe hypovolemia, dehydration, and hypotension, percutaneous vascular access may be difficult or impossible. Surgical cutdown allows direct visualization of the vein for ease of catheter placement. Vascular cutdown is usually performed in emergent situations. Although sterile technique should be maintained at all times, the risk of introducing bacteria into the patient's vessel is great. For this reason, cut-down should be performed in emergencies, and then the catheter changed to a percutaneous catheter as soon as the patient's volume and blood pressure have been normalized.

Supplies Needed

Electric clippers and blades
Antimicrobial scrub solution
Sterile gauze 4- × 4-sponges
Sterile gloves
Sterile surgical pack
   Scalpel handle and number 11 scalpel blade
   Field towels
   Towel clamps
   Tissue/thumb forceps
   Mosquito hemostats
   Mettzenbaum scissors
   Needle holders
3–0 absorbable suture
14- to 18-gauge venocath or over-the-needle peripheral catheter
Heparinized saline flush solution
T-port connector or male adapter
2-inch Kling bandaging material
1-inch white tape
Elastikon® bandaging material

Indications

Catheterization of vessel in patients with extreme hypotension, peripheral vasoconstriction, or obesity
Infusion of crystalloid or colloid fluids
Infusion of blood products
Infusion of drugs
Obtain blood samples

Contraindications

Abrasion, burn, or pyoderma over catheter site
Direct percutaneous catheterization is possible

 Video available online

Go to www.wiley.com/go/hackett to view a video of this procedure.

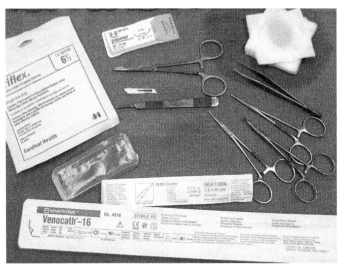

Fig. 1.64. Supplies needed for vascular cutdown.

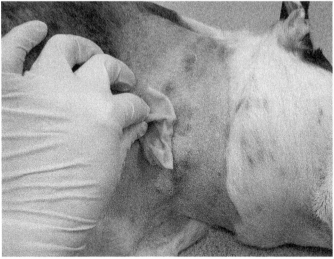

Fig. 1.65. After clipping the fur and then aseptically scrubbing the clipped area, drape the surgical site with sterile field towels.

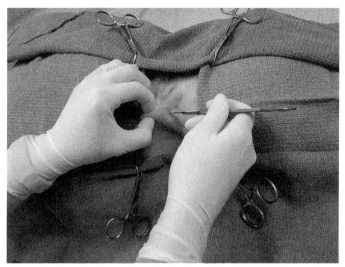

Fig. 1.66. Tent skin over site of proposed vascular catheterization. Incise the skin using a number 11 scalpel blade.

Helpful hint: Gently move the skin away from the vein to avoid cutting the vessel.

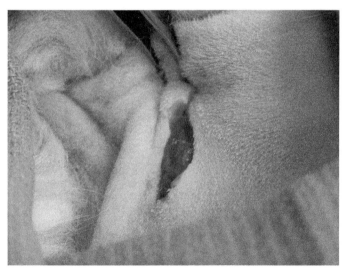

Fig. 1.67. Visualize the vessel under the skin incision.

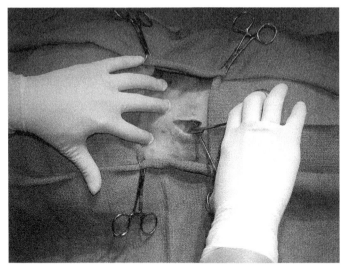

Fig. 1.68. Bluntly dissect the fascia overlying the vessel using a curved mosquito forceps.

Helpful hint: Make sure that all of fascia is dissected away from vessel, or else attempts at placing the catheter into the vessel will be difficult.

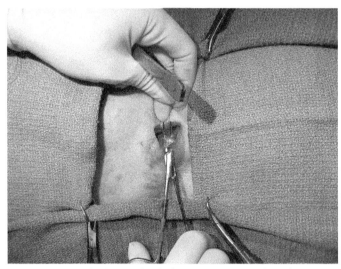

Fig. 1.69. Insert curved hemostats under the vessel and raise the vessel to the skin surface.

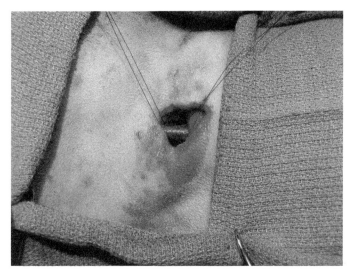

Fig. 1.70. Place two separate absorbable stay sutures securely with mosquito hemostats to raise the vessel to the level and parallel with the skin surface.

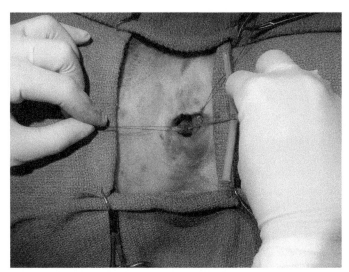

Fig. 1.71. With the vessel raised and parallel to the skin surface, gently puncture the vessel with the needle, and insert the catheter.

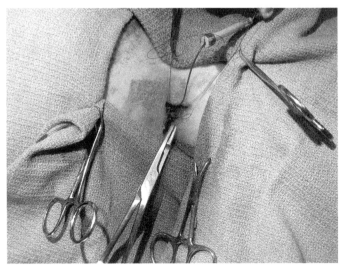

Fig. 1.72. Gently tie the stay sutures, occluding the vessel.

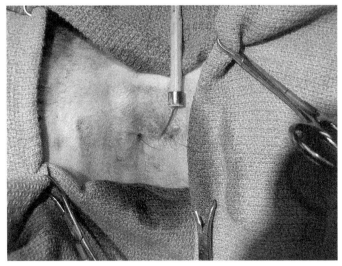

Fig. 1.73. Suture the skin overlying the point of catheter insertion. Bandage in place as with a percutaneously placed catheter. The vessel will remain ligated. Collateral circulation will suffice. If the vessel is not occluded, there will be too much hemorrhage.

Helpful hint: This catheter can be removed when a percutaneous catheter can be placed.

INTRAOSSEOUS CATHETERIZATION

Introduction

Intraosseous catheterization is often necessary in pediatric small animal patients and exotic species when vascular access is impossible. Any fluid, including blood products and parenteral nutrition, that can be infused into a peripheral or central catheter can be infused through an intraosseous catheter. Although intraosseous catheters are well-tolerated, the catheter or needle traverses the periosteum and intraosseous catheters are somewhat uncomfortable; they should be changed to a venous catheter whenever possible.

Supplies Needed

Electric clippers and blades
Antimicrobial scrub solution
2% lidocaine
1- to 3-ml syringe and 22-gauge needle
3-ml syringe with heparinized flush solution
Number 11 scalpel blade
16- to 18-gauge bone marrow needles or spinal needles with stylette
20- to 22-gauge hypodermic needles
1/2-inch to 1-inch white tape
T-port or male adapter flushed with heparinized saline
3–0 nylon suture
Optional supplies: EZ-IO® device and catheter

Indications

Infusion of crystalloid and synthetic colloid fluids, and blood products
Infusion of drugs
Infusion of parenteral nutrition
Vascular access is impossible

Contraindications

Pyoderma or abrasion over site of intraosseous catheter placement
Ambulatory patients, as catheter can become dislodged
Intravenous catheterization is possible

 Video available online

Go to www.wiley.com/go/hackett to view a video of this procedure.

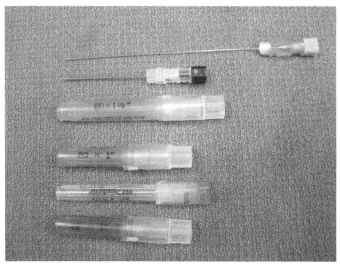

Fig. 1.74. Supplies needed for intraosseous catheterization.

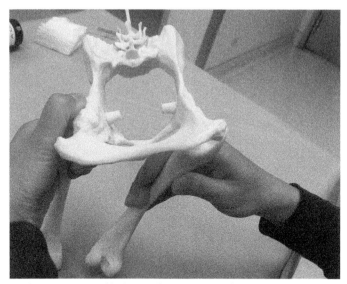

Fig. 1.75. Abduct the femur so that the stifle is away from the body. This allows the sciatic nerve to move out of the way of catheter placement.

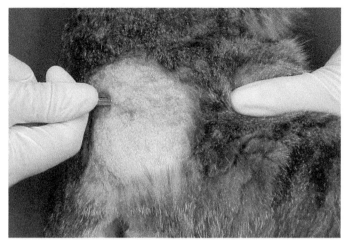

Fig. 1.76. Palpate the greater (major) trochanter of the femur. The trochanteric fossa drops off medially from the greater trochanter. Insert the needle through the skin after placing a bleb of 2% lidocaine into the level of the periosteum. Walk the tip of the needle medially off the greater trochanter into trochanteric fossa. Once the needle is against bone at the bottom of the trochanteric fossa, push the needle in parallel with the femur. Then use a simultaneous twisting and pushing motion to seat the catheter into the medullary cavity. In larger animals, you can make a stab incision with a number 11 scalpel blade before needle placement to prevent tissue drag.

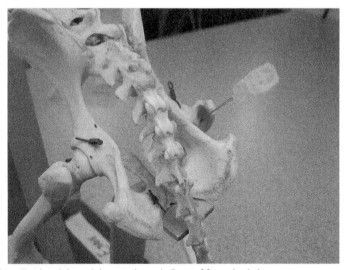

Fig. 1.77. Spinal needle placed through intertrochanteric fossa of femur in skeleton.

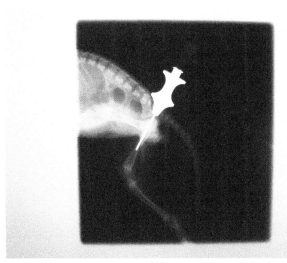

Fig. 1.78. Once the needle is in the correct position, infuse a small amount of saline. The saline should flow freely. Check catheter placement with a lateral and AP radiograph.

Helpful hint: If you place a catheter using a hypodermic needle, the needle can sometimes become clogged with bone debris. If this occurs, remove the needle and replace an identical needle in the same hole.

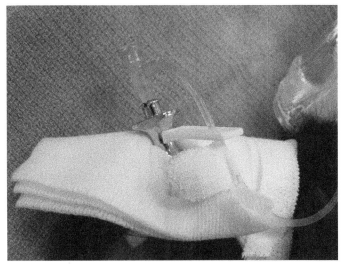

Fig. 1.79. Secure a piece of half- or 1-inch tape around the hub of the needle and male adapter, and tape around body. Alternatively, you can make wings of tape and suture to the skin at the base of the catheter hub.

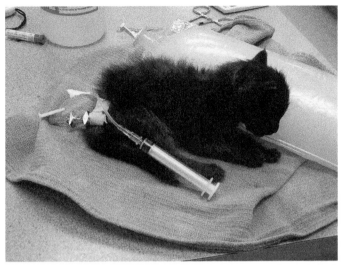

Fig. 1.80. Patients will tolerate the intraosseous (IO) catheter quite well. Place the patient in lateral recumbency. Mild sedation is usually necessary to place IO catheters in the humerus. Clip and aseptically scrub the proximal humerus cranially, over the greater tubercle, then palpate the greater tubercle, on the anterior portion of the proximal humerus.

Helpful hint: As soon as the patient is ambulatory or vascular access can be obtained, place an intravenous catheter and remove the intraosseous catheter. Helpful hint: It is often necessary to flex and extend the shoulder several times to palpate the scapulohumeral joint, then the greater tubercle of the humerus.

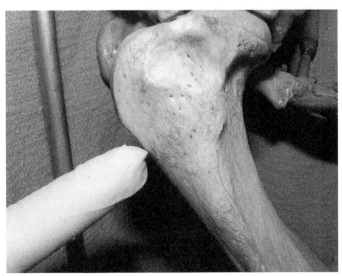

Fig. 1.81. Greater tubercle of the humerus on skeleton.

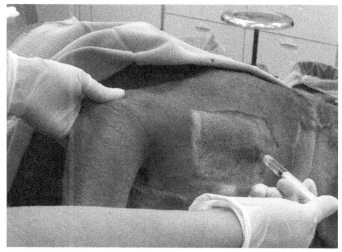

Fig. 1.82. Infiltrate through the skin and underlying fascia to the level of the periosteum with 2% lidocaine (1 mg/kg).

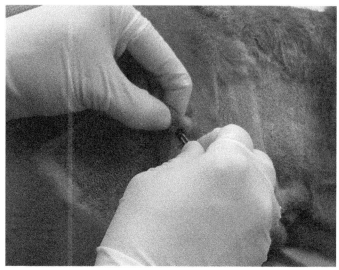

Fig. 1.83. Make a small nick incision through the skin with a number 11 scalpel blade.

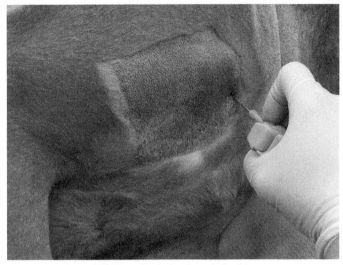

Fig. 1.84. Insert the IO catheter/Jamshidi® IO needle device through the skin.

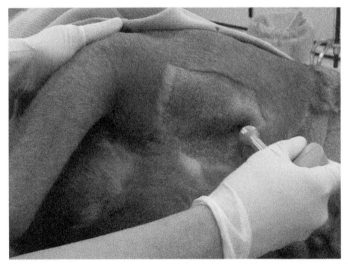

Fig. 1.85. Bend the limb such that the distal humerus/elbow is almost at a 90° angle to the scapulohumeral joint. Place the nondominant hand on the elbow, and the dominant hand on the IO catheter. Push the IO catheter into the greater tubercle of the humerus, pushing with a simultaneous twisting motion.

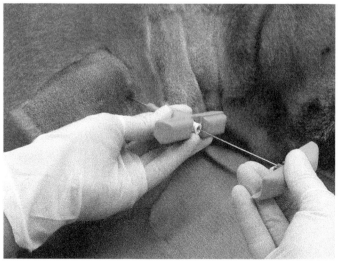

Fig. 1.86. Once the catheter is seated in the marrow cavity, remove the internal stylet.

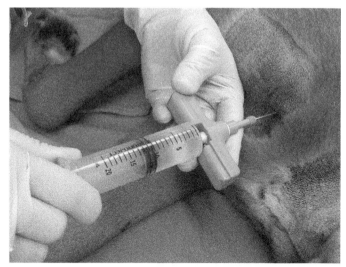

Fig. 1.87. Flush the catheter with sterile 0.9% saline. If seated properly, the flush will be easy, with minimal resistance.

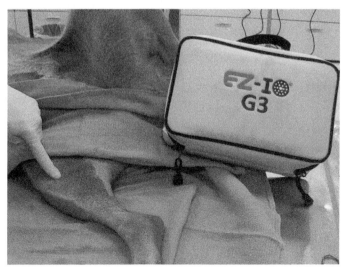

Fig. 1.88. In veterinary patients, the medial aspect of the proximal tibia is the most easily accessible, and has minimal subcutaneous tissue to interfere with placement of the EZ-IO® catheter.

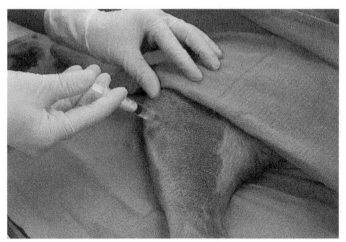

Fig. 1.89. Clip and aseptically scrub the medial aspect of the proximal tibia. Infiltrate the area with 2% lidocaine (1 mg/kg) from the level of the skin to the periosteum.

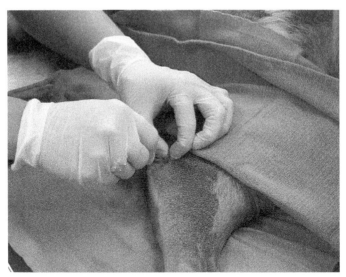

Fig. 1.90. Make a small nick incision in the skin, through the anesthetized area, with a number 15 or 11 scalpel blade.

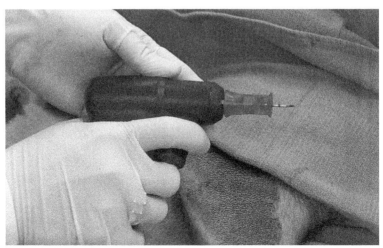

Fig. 1.91. The EZ-IO® device is essentially a drill equipped with a disposable metal intraosseous catheter.

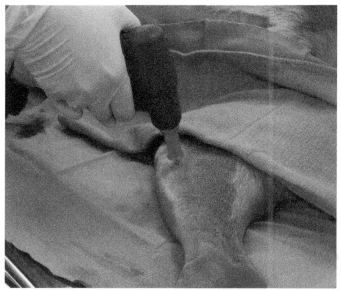

Fig. 1.92. Insert the IO device through the nick incision in the skin, and push while simultaneously engaging the drill apparatus, to allow penetration of the IO catheter into the proximal tibia.

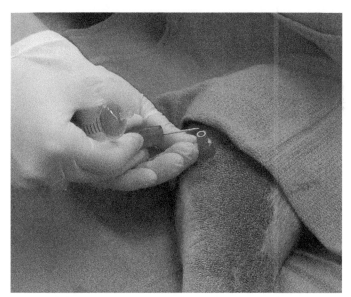

Fig. 1.93. Once the catheter is firmly inserted into the proximal tibia, remove the inner cannula.

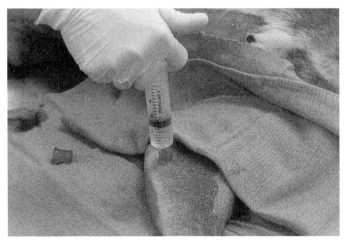
Fig. 1.94. Flush the IO catheter with sterile 0.9% saline. The catheter should flush easily, with minimal resistance, if inserted properly.

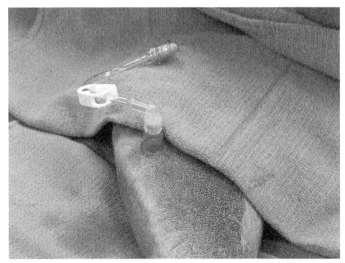
Fig. 1.95. Attach a luer-lock T-port to the IO catheter. The catheter is ready for use.

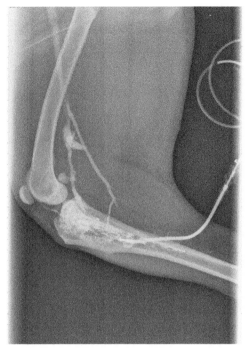

Fig. 1.96. Radiograph with iodinated contrast material demonstrating immediate entry into peripheral circulation through the intraosseous catheter. Photo courtesy of Dr. Steve Mensack.

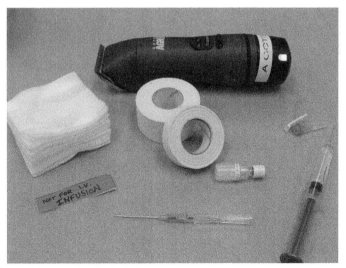

Fig. 1.97. Supplies needed for arterial catheterization.

ARTERIAL CATHETERIZATION

Introduction

Arterial catheterization is a technique that is useful in nonambulatory critically ill small animal patients. Arterial catheters should be placed when repeated arterial blood samples are required, such as in patients with pulmonary or cardiac disease when monitoring of oxygenation and ventilation is desirable. Arterial catheters also can be used for continuous invasive blood pressure monitoring. Arterial catheters are commonly placed in the dorsal pedal, femoral, coccygeal, and auricular arteries.

Supplies Needed

Electric clippers
Electric clipper blades
Antimicrobial scrub solution
Over-the-needle catheters (20-, 22-, and 24-gauge)
1/2- and 1-inch white adhesive tape
T-port or luer-lock male adapters (flushed with heparinized saline)
Cotton balls
3-ml syringes with heparinized saline
Permanent marker to label catheter
Stickers "Not for IV infusion"

Indications

Measurement of direct arterial blood pressure
Obtain blood samples for blood gas analyses

Contraindications

Abrasions, burns, pyoderma over site of catheter placement
Thromboembolic disease or hypercoagulability
Coagulopathy
Ambulatory patients that will disconnect catheter
Never to be used for blood sample, drug, or fluid infusion

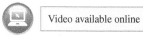 Video available online

Go to www.wiley.com/go/hackett to view a video of this procedure.

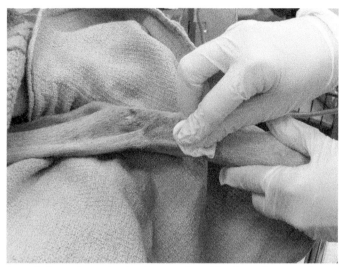

Fig. 1.98. Clip and aseptically scrub over the site of proposed arterial catheter placement. Common insertion sites include the dorsal pedal, femoral, or auricular arteries.

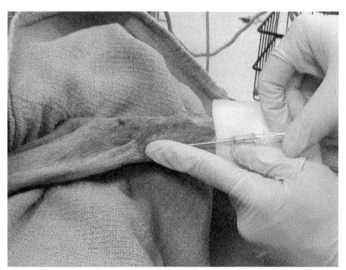

Fig. 1.99. Insert the needle through the skin at a 30° to 45° angle. Once the needle is under the skin, palpate the arterial pulse and direct the needle into the artery using very small, blunt movements. Watch carefully for a flash of blood in the hub of the stylette. Unlike venous catheterization, there is no "pop" felt as the catheter passes through the thick vessel wall.

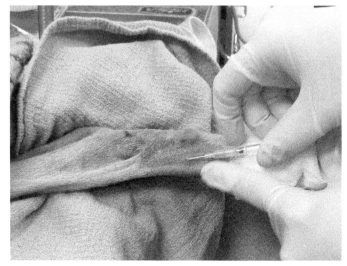

Fig. 1.100. Once the blood is in the catheter hub, gently push the catheter off of the stylette into the artery.

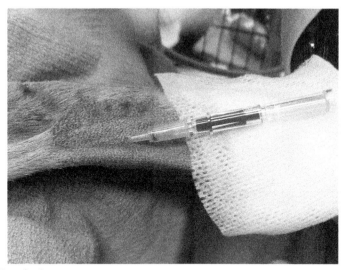

Fig. 1.101a. Catheter in place.

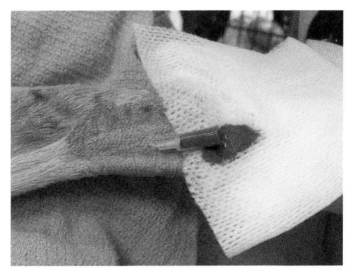

Fig. 1.101b. Once the catheter is in place, blood will flow freely. Flush the catheter immediately with heparinized saline and secure it in place as with any other catheter.

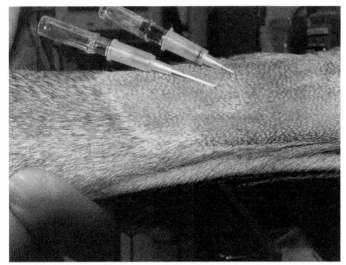

Fig. 1.102. If the catheter won't feed easily, direct it so that it is parallel with the artery. If you cannot feed the catheter, keep the catheter in place and start again proximally to the point of original catheter attempt. If you remove the original catheter, a hematoma will form, preventing further attempts into the same artery.

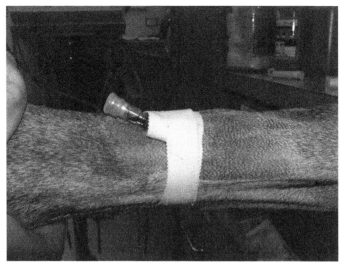

Fig. 1.103. Tape the catheter around the hub and limb with a half-inch length of white adhesive tape.

Helpful hint: Make sure that the catheter hub and skin are completely dry, so that the tape will securely attach itself to the catheter hub and the catheter will not spin around, or else the catheter will not remain in place and will pull out of the vessel.

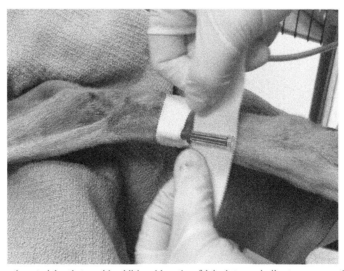

Fig. 1.104. Secure the arterial catheter with additional lengths of 1-inch tape, similar to venous catheters.

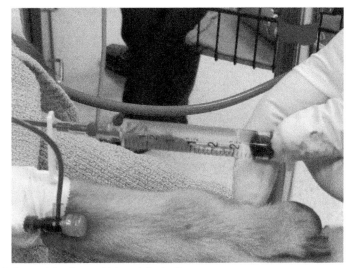

Fig. 1.105. Flush the arterial catheter with heparinized saline.

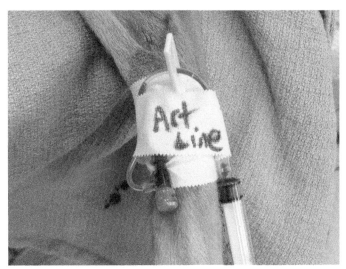

Fig. 1.106. Label the arterial catheter prominently with "Not for IV infusion."

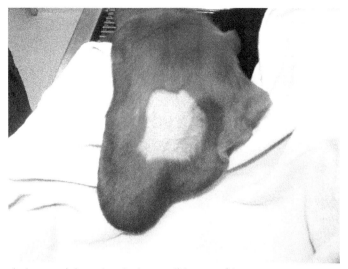

Fig. 1.107. The auricular artery is located on the dorsomedial aspect of the ear.

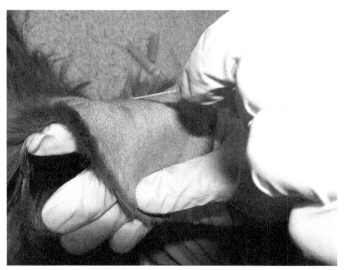

Fig. 1.108. Clip and aseptically scrub the ear. Fold the ear tip over the fingers of your non-dominant hand. The artery is located in the middle. The catheter can be inserted directly into the artery.

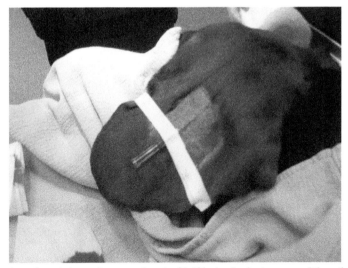

Fig. 1.109. Once the catheter is inserted, secure a length of half-inch adhesive tape around the catheter hub, and then around the ear.

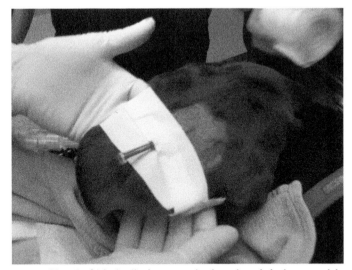

Fig. 1.110. Secure a second length of 1-inch adhesive tape under the catheter hub, then around the ear.

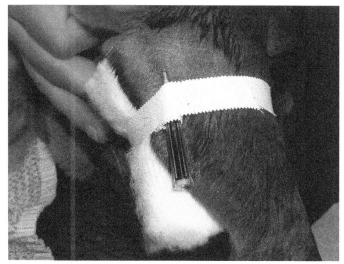

Fig. 1.111. Finally, secure the ear around a roll of gauze or cotton, then bandage in place.

REFERENCES

Beal MW, Hughes D. Vascular access: Theory and techniques in the small animal emergency patient. *Clin Tech Sm Anim Pract* 15(2):101–109, 2000.

Hughes D, Beal MW. Emergency vascular access. *Vet Clin North Amer Small Anim* 30(3):491–507, 2000.

Otto CM, Kaufman GM, Crowe DT. Intraosseous infusion of fluids and therapeutics. *Compend Contin Educ Pract Vet* 11:421–430, 1989.

Poundstone M. Intraosseous infusion of fluids in small animals. *Vet Tech* 13:407–412, 1992.

Sacchetti A. Large-bore infusion catheters (Seldinger technique for vascular access). In: Roberts JR, Hedges JR (Eds): Clinical Procedures in Emergency Medicine. Philadelphia: WB Saunders. pp. 289–293, 1985.

CHAPTER 2

Nutritional Support and Orogastric Lavage

INTRODUCTION

Nutritional support of the critically ill patient is important to providing necessary proteins, carbohydrates, and lipids for energy and repair processes in a variety of illnesses. The placement of an enteral feeding tube for nutritional supplementation is preferred and should be considered in any patient that has a functioning gastrointestinal tract and is not vomiting. This chapter describes the placement and maintenance of a variety of enteral feeding devices, including nasoesophageal, nasogastric, esophagostomy, and jejunostomy tubes.

NASOESOPHAGEAL AND NASOGASTRIC TUBES

Introduction

Nasoesophageal and nasogastric feeding tubes should be considered in any patient for short-term enteral nutritional support when the patient either cannot or will not voluntarily eat and has no known esophageal disorder and is not vomiting. Specialized veterinary liquid enteral diets are commercially available for use with nasoesophageal and nasogastric tubes. In addition to providing enteral nutrition, nasoesophageal and nasogastric tubes can also be used to suction air and fluid from the esophagus and stomach in patients with severe ileus.

Supplies Needed

Needle holders
Proparacaine
Nonabsorbable suture (3–0)
5 to 10 French Argyle infant feeding tube or red rubber catheter

Veterinary Emergency and Critical Care Procedures, Second Edition. Timothy B. Hackett and Elisa M. Mazzaferro.
© 2012 John Wiley & Sons, Inc. Published 2012 by John Wiley & Sons, Inc.

Permanent marker
Elizabethan collar

Indications

Short-term enteral nutrition in patients that are inappetant
Suctioning of gastric fluid or air in cases of severe ileus

Contraindications

Nasopharyngeal trauma
Vomiting
Esophageal reflux
Regurgitation
Esophageal strictures or foreign bodies
Megaesophagus
Thrombocytopenia
Recumbent or unconscious patients

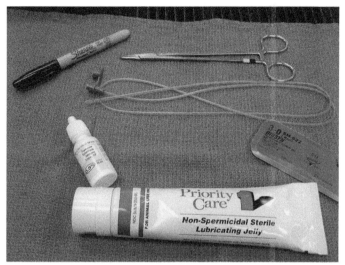

Fig. 2.1. Supplies needed for a nasoesophageal or nasogastric tube include an infant feeding tube, 3–0 nonabsorbable suture, topical proparacaine, permanent marker, sterile lubricating jelly, and needle holders.

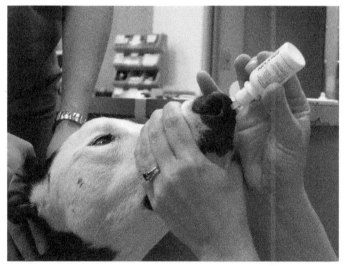

Fig. 2.2. Tilt the patient's head upward toward the ceiling and place several drops of topical proparacaine into the nostril.

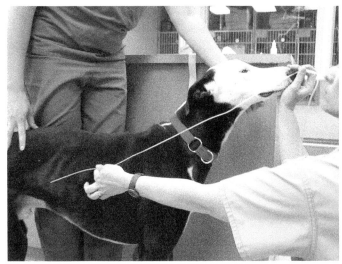

Fig. 2.3. Measure the feeding tube to the level of the carina (nasoesophageal) or last rib (nasogastric) and mark the tube with a permanent marker.

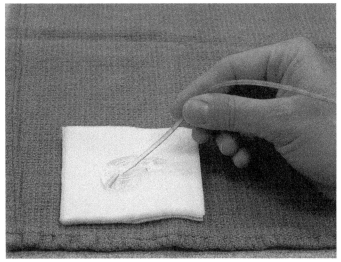

Fig. 2.4. Lubricate the tip of the tube with sterile lubricant jelly.

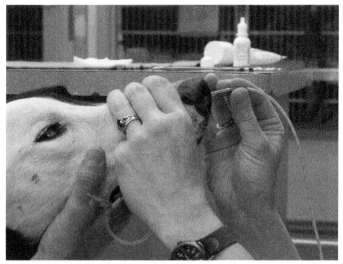

Fig. 2.5. Grasp the dog's muzzle and gently and briskly insert the tube ventrally and medially.

Helpful hint: Hold onto the tube as close to the patient's muzzle as possible, to prevent the patient from sneezing the tube back out at you. Push the patient's nose toward the ceiling when passing the tube to extend the neck. The patient should swallow the tube.

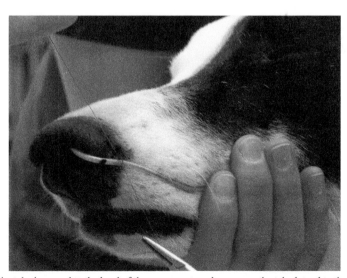

Fig. 2.6. Once the tube is passed to the level of the permanent marker, secure the tube lateral to the nostril with a suture or surgical staple.

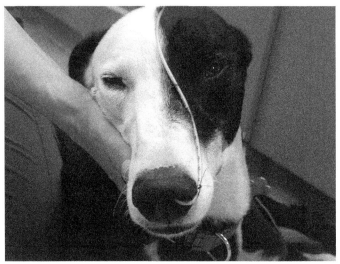

Fig. 2.7. Secure the tube lateral to the eye, or medial to the eye, and to the top of the head with sutures or surgical staples. Take care to avoid the patient's whiskers.

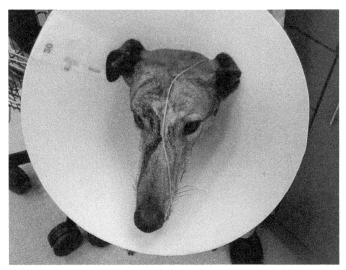

Fig. 2.8. Place an Elizabethan collar on the patient to prevent tube displacement.

Helpful hint: If the tube is bothersome to the patient and the patient is sneezing, apply more topical anesthetic as needed to minimize patient discomfort. Check the placement of the tube with a lateral thoracic radiograph. If the tube does not have a radiopaque marker, add a small amount of iodinated contrast material. Once placement has been confirmed, the tube can be used immediately. It is advisable to start all feedings with 5 to 10 cc of water. If the patient has accidentally aspirated the tube into the trachea, fluid will elicit a cough. The tube position should be rechecked. Upon tube removal, make sure that the tube is kinked well and then pulled briskly, to prevent fluid from entering the trachea and lungs.

ESOPHAGOSTOMY TUBES

Introduction

An esophagostomy tube should be considered whenever a patient is inappetant because it either voluntarily will not or cannot eat (i.e., severe maxillofacial trauma, neoplasia or mass effects, inappetance). Esophagostomy tubes are simple to place, require minimal equipment, and can be used immediately. An esophagostomy tube is contraindicated in patients that cannot protect their airway, are vomiting or regurgitating, or have functional or mechanical esophageal abnormalities such as megaesophagus or strictures.

Supplies Needed

Surgical instruments
   Number 10 scalpel blade
   Scalpel handle
   Needle holders
   Mayo scissors
   Rochester carmalt
   Nonabsorbable suture (variety of sizes, depending on size of tube and patient)
Permanent marker
Electric clippers and blades
Antimicrobial scrub
Christmas tree adapter
Bandage material
   Gauze, 4-×4-inch squares
   Cotton roll gauze
   Kling
   Elastikon® or Vetrap™
Red rubber or other tube for E tube
Optional supplies: Braun esophagostomy insertion device

Indications

Inappetance
Maxillofacial trauma
Severe dental disease
Orofacial, pharyngeal masses

Contraindications

Vomiting
Regurgitation
Esophageal stricture or foreign body
Megaesophagus
Conditions in which patient cannot protect its airway
Severe cough
Pneumonia

 | Video available online

Go to www.wiley.com/go/hackett to view a video of this procedure.

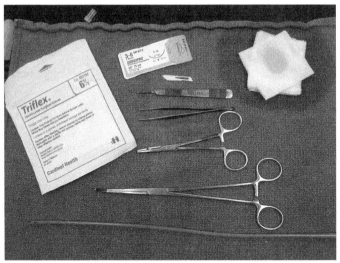

Fig. 2.9. Materials needed for placement of an esophagostomy tube include a red rubber tube (10 to 20 French depending on size of patient), number 10 scalpel blade and handle, Rochester carmalt, Mayo scissors, needle holder, permanent marker, non-absorbable suture, electric clippers and blade, antimicrobial scrub, and a Christmas tree adapter.

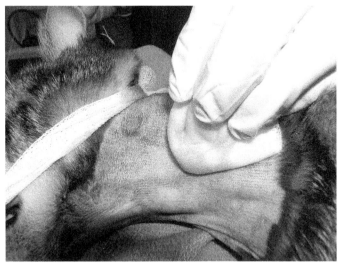

Fig. 2.10. Anesthetize and intubate the patient. Place the patient in right lateral recumbency, and clip the neck from the ramus of the mandible caudally to the thoracic inlet and dorsally and ventrally to midline. Aseptically scrub the clipped area.

Helpful hint: If the patient is intubated, there is only one tube into which you can possibly insert your esophagostomy tube.

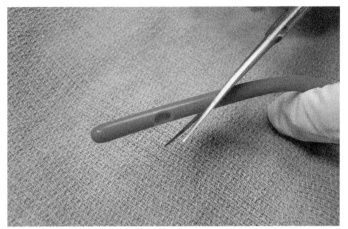

Fig. 2.11. Cut the distal end of the red rubber tube on a diagonal proximal to the holes in the tube. This will increase the diameter through which food is passed, decreasing the risk of tube occlusion.

Helpful hint: Make sure that the cut edges of the distal end of the tube are not sharp to prevent esophageal irritation.

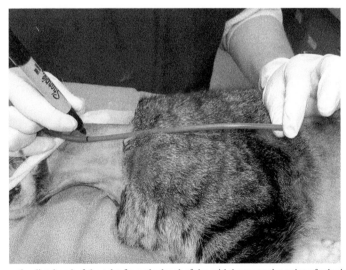

Fig. 2.12. Measure the distal end of the tube from the level of the mid thorax to the point of tube insertion in the lateral cervical region. Mark the tube at the point of insertion with the permanent marker.

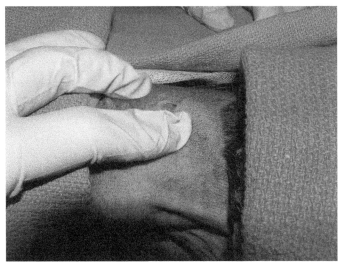

Fig. 2.13. With the patient anesthetized, drape the clipped area with sterile field towels secured with towel clamps. Gently pull the tongue rostrally, and insert a Rochester carmalt into the mouth and down the throat, bringing the tips of the carmalt laterally to the skin at the level of mid-cervical region. You should be able to palpate the tips of the carmalt under the skin with your fingertips.

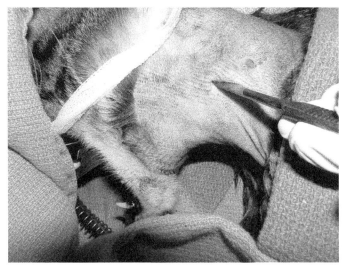

Fig. 2.14. Open the tips of the carmalt and make a stab incision with the scalpel blade through the skin and underlying fascia, into the esophagus. You should be able to push the tips of the carmalt laterally through the edges of the skin incision.

Helpful hint: In some cases, it may be necessary to gently incise the esophagus over the tips of the carmalt. Make sure to keep the tips of the carmalt in sight, so as to create only one hole.

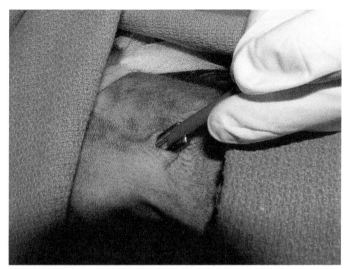

Fig. 2.15. Grasp the distal end of the red rubber tube and clamp it in the tips of the carmalt.

Helpful hint: At this point, it is easy to also grasp tissue in the mouth or esophagus in the hinges of the Carmalt. This will prevent you from easily bringing the tube forward.

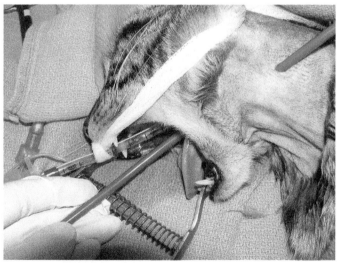

Fig. 2.16. Pull the distal end of the red rubber tube rostrally out the front of the mouth. The proximal end of the tube will be facing caudally at this point.

Helpful hint: If you are not able to pull the tube forward easily, make sure that you do not have tissue caught in the hinges of the carmalt, and make sure that the red rubber tube or carmalt is not wrapped around the tie-gauze of the endotracheal tube.

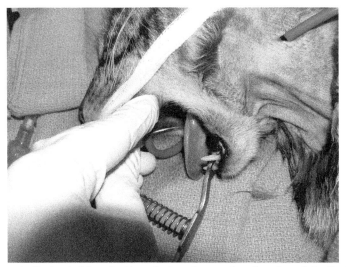

Fig. 2.17. Unclamp the distal end of the red rubber tube from the carmalt, and gently push the distal end caudally. Use your fingers or the carmalt to push the distal end of the tube down the esophagus.

Helpful hint: Make sure that the patient is well-anesthetized before attempting this step because he can clamp onto your fingers with stimulation in his mouth.

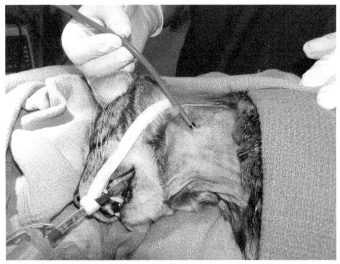

Fig. 2.18. Once the tube is in place, the proximal end of the tube will "flip" rostrally toward the front of the patient. At this point, gently twist the tube to make sure it is in the correct place.

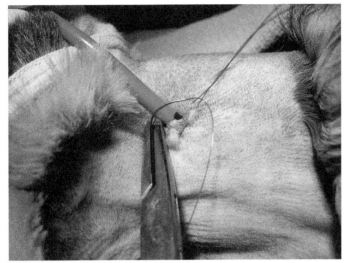

Fig. 2.19. Place a holding suture, or loose purse-string suture, around the entrance of the tube site, leaving the ends long. Place a finger-trap suture around the base of the tube, where the tube enters the skin.

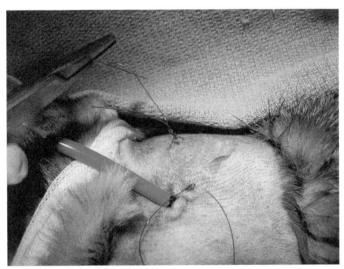

Fig. 2.20. Some criticalists advocate using a wide suture, scraping the periosteum of the atlas to secure the mid portion of the tube in place to the wing of the atlas.

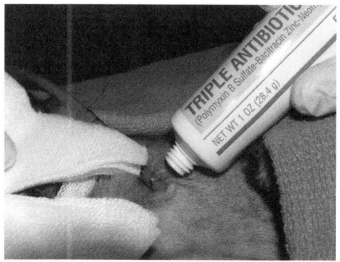

Fig. 2.21. Place antimicrobial ointment over the entry site, and then loosely bandage the tube in place. Check the tube for erythema and drainage on a daily basis.

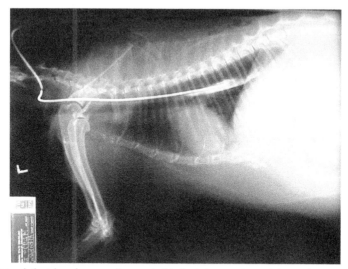

Fig. 2.22. Radiograph the tube using a small amount of iodinated contrast material, to make sure tube is in place, before using. When correct placement has been confirmed, the tube can be used immediately.

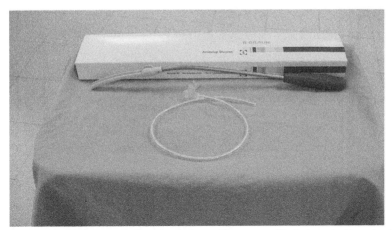

Fig. 2.23. The Braun esophagostomy tube insertion device, and instruments like it, is a valuable tool to help facilitate placement of esophagostomy tubes in small animals (cats and small dogs).

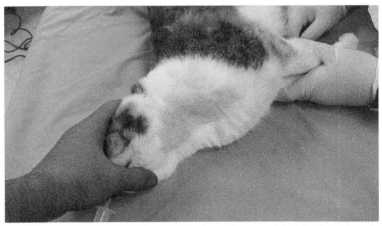

Fig. 2.24. The anesthetized, intubated cat is placed in lateral recumbency, and the left side of the neck clipped and aseptically scrubbed as previously described.

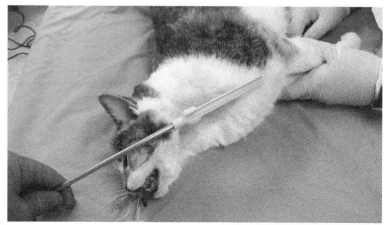

Fig. 2.25. The esophagostomy tube insertion device is measured against the lateral body wall.

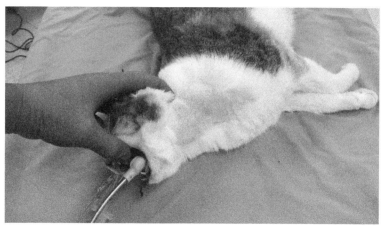

Fig. 2.26. The insertion device is placed into the cat's mouth, down the esophagus.

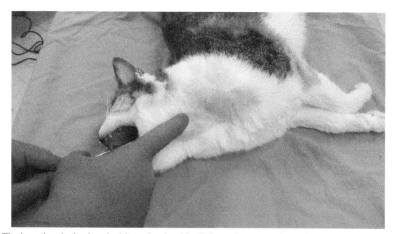

Fig. 2.27. The insertion device is palpable under the skin. Palpate the groove in the insertion device.

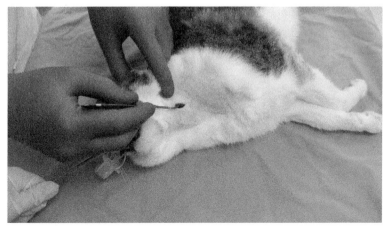

Fig. 2.28. Make an incision through the skin and into the esophagus, using a number 10 scalpel blade.

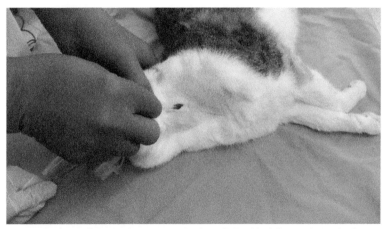

Fig. 2.29. Insert the distal end of the esophagostomy tube through the skin defect, and start feeding caudally down the esophagus.

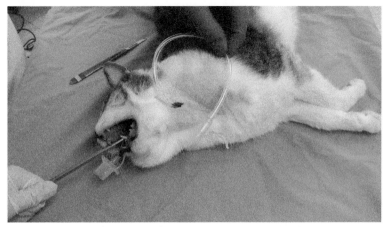

Fig. 2.30. Once the tube is inserted to the level of the carina, it can be sutured in place.

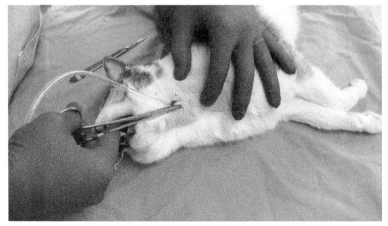

Fig. 2.31. Place a purse-string suture around the tube entrance site with nonabsorbable suture.

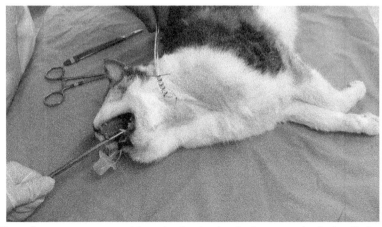

Fig. 2.32. Place a finger-trap suture around then tube, then bandage in place as previously described.

OROGASTRIC LAVAGE

Introduction

Orogastric lavage is an important means of removal of ingesta from the stomach of animals that have ingested toxins or excessive food, as in the case of food bloat. The technique should be performed after induction of general anesthesia, endotracheal intubation with a cuffed endotracheal tube, and maintenance on gas or intravenous anesthesia and oxygen supplementation. Orogastric lavage should be considered whenever an animal is not able to vomit, or if induction of emesis is contraindicated in a patient with neurologic abnormalities and cannot protect its airway.

Supplies Needed

Orogastric tube or 60-ml syringe
Two buckets
Warm tap water
Lavage pump
Mouth gag
Tape or permanent marker

Indications

Removal of toxins from stomach
Removal of food from stomach
Gastric decompression

Contraindications

Should not be performed in awake, non-intubated animals
that cannot protect their airway
Gastric perforation
Removal of caustic substances

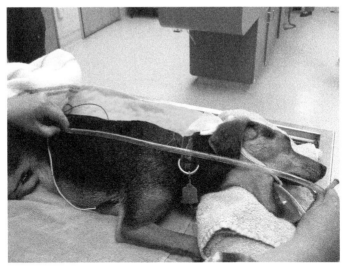

Fig. 2.33. Place the patient in sternal or lateral recumbency with a cuffed endotracheal tube in place. Measure the orogastric tube from the tip of the nose to the last rib.

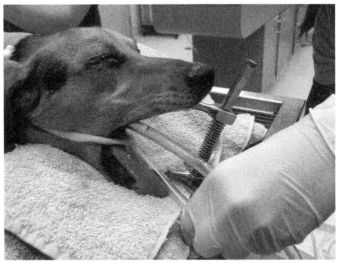

Fig. 2.34. Insert the lubricated tube through the mouth, to the level of the last rib, into the stomach.

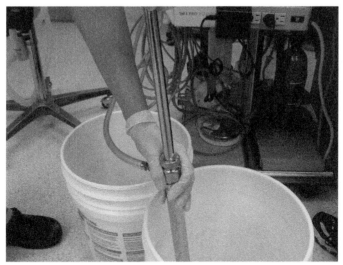

Fig. 2.35. Attach the distal end of the orogastric tube to the lavage pump, and instill tap water warmed to body temperature into the stomach. Monitor the patient for respiratory distress or excessive abdominal distension.

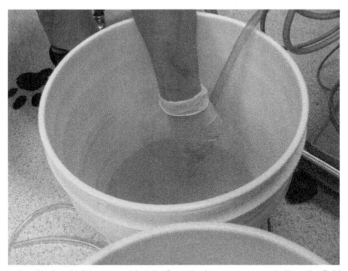

Fig. 2.36. Separate the distal end of the orogastric tube from the lavage pump, and allow the fluid and gastric contents to flow into a second collection bucket. Save specimens for later analysis for toxins, if necessary.

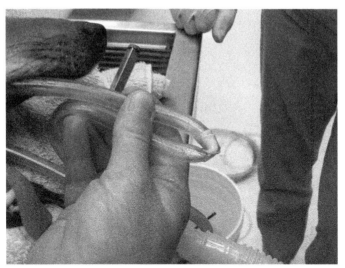

Fig. 2.37. Once the effluent fluid is clear, and the stomach has been emptied of its contents, kink the tube tightly at the level of the mouth and quickly remove. Kinking the tube will help prevent backflow of gastric contents and fluid into the esophagus or lungs during tube removal.

JEJUNOSTOMY TUBE

Introduction

Whenever any portion of the gastrointestinal tract can be used for enteral nutrition, it should be considered. Placement of a jejunostomy tube at the time of abdominal surgery should be considered in any patient that is inappetant, vomiting, or has a portion of the proximal gastrointestinal tract (i.e., esophagus, stomach, pancreas, or duodenum) that needs to be rested or bypassed due to disease or need for healing. Jejunostomy tubes can be used 24 hours after placement, and should be left in place for a minimum of seven days before removal to prevent leakage from the site and peritonitis. Only fluids should be administered through the jejunostomy tube (J tube), because the small luminal size can easily become clogged and obstructed. Placement of the J tube will not prevent vomiting.

Supplies

Number 11 scalpel blade
Straight hemostat forceps
Argyle feeding tube or red rubber catheter (5 to 10 French depending on patient size)
4–0 or 3–0 absorbable suture
4–0 or 3–0 nonabsorbable suture

Indications

Provision of enteral nutrition in a patient that is vomiting or must have proximal gastrointestinal tract bypassed

Contraindications

Severe hypoalbuminemia
Peritonitis
Jejunal disease

Potential Complications

Inadvertent premature removal of tube before seal has occurred
Leakage of jejunal contents into abdomen
Peritonitis
Oral displacement of tube
Vomiting
Tube clog/malfunction

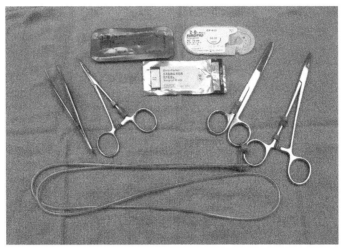

Fig. 2.38. Supplies needed for placement of a jejunostomy tube.

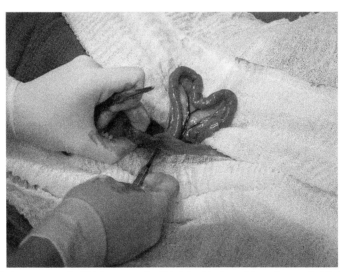

Fig. 2.39. Exteriorize segment of mid-jejunum, and pull to lateral body wall to make sure that there will not be tension once secured in place.

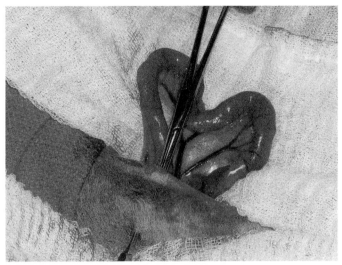

Fig. 2.40. Make a stab incision through the skin on the ventrolateral abdominal wall. Once the scalpel is through the body wall, clamp it with a straight hemostat forceps, and pull the hemostat through the hole made by the scalpel.

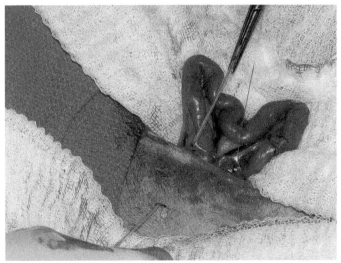

Fig. 2.41. With the hemostat, pull the tip of a red rubber or Argyle feeding tube through the body wall, into the peritoneal cavity.

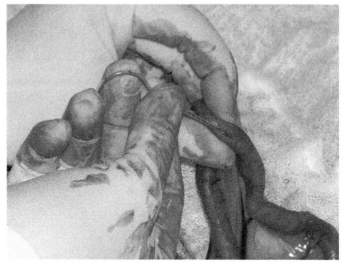

Fig. 2.42. Make a 1- to 1.5-cm incision through the serosa to the submucosa on the antimesenteric border of the jejunum.

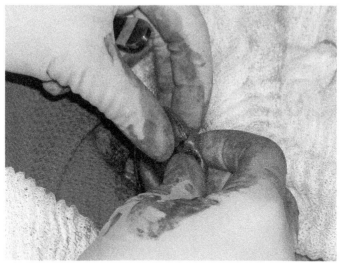

Fig. 2.43. Tunnel at least 10 cm to 12 cm of the jejunostomy tube through the submucosa into the jejunal lumen, pushing in an aboral direction.

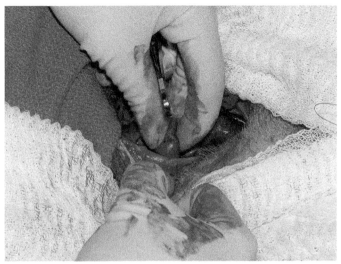

Fig. 2.44. Attach the jejunal segment to the ventrolateral body wall using an absorbable purse-string suture, securing the jejunum to peritoneum in at least four places.

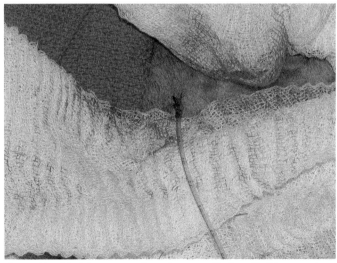

Fig. 2.45. Secure the outside of the jejunostomy tube to the external body wall with a second purse-string, then finger-trap suture using nonabsorbable suture.

PARENTERAL NUTRITION

Introduction

Injured or critically ill animals are at high risk for malnutrition and its subsequent complications. Critically ill animals will lose lean body mass when they are not given sufficient calories. This loss reduces the animal's strength, immune function, wound healing, and overall survival. Therefore, it is important to provide nutritional support to animals that are not willing or able to eat adequate amounts orally.

Calculating Energy Requirements

The patient's resting energy requirement (RER) is used as the initial estimate of a hospitalized patient's calorie requirements. Further adjustments are then made on the basis of the patient's response to feeding, body weight, and changes in the underlying condition. RER is rarely exceeded for hospitalized patients. With the exception of sepsis, most critically ill patients have caloric needs very close to RER.

The RER in kilocalories/day is 70 (weight in kg). For animals between 2 and 30 kg, the following equation also can be used:

$$30 \text{ (weight in kg)} + 70.$$

Administering Parenteral Nutrition

Parenteral nutrition (PN) should never be viewed as an emergency procedure. Patients should be hemodynamically stable with major electrolyte disorders corrected. Both total parenteral nutrition (TPN) and partial parenteral nutrition (PPN) require a dedicated catheter. An exception to this is when multi-lumen catheters are used. In this case, one lumen of the catheter is dedicated to parenteral nutrition while the other lumen(s) can be used for other purposes.

TPN should be started gradually (50% of total requirements on day 1, 75% to 100% of total requirements on day 2). Therefore, it will take two to three days to reach the animal's total nutritional requirements. In most cases, PPN can be started full strength. Parenteral nutrition should be administered by continuous rate infusion via a fluid pump over 24 hours. When parenteral nutrition is administered, any other intravenous fluids that the patient is receiving must be adjusted accordingly to avoid volume overload. The PN and fluid line should not be disconnected except when changing to a new bag.

Once the patient is able to eat, it should be offered food regularly to assess its appetite. When the patient is voluntarily consuming more than 60% of its energy requirements, TPN can be gradually decreased over a period of four to eight hours. Tapering of PPN is unnecessary. Any partially used or unused solutions from a patient should be discarded.

Potential Complications and Monitoring

Potential complications of parenteral nutrition include metabolic disturbances (e.g., hyperglycemia, electrolyte abnormalities, hypertriglyceridemia), mechanical problems of the catheter and lines, and septic complications. Careful monitoring is important to reduce the risk of complications. At least the following should be measured daily in all animals receiving parenteral nutrition: heart rate, respiratory rate, temperature, attitude, body weight, catheter site, and glucose. All blood tubes should be examined for gross lipemia. Monitoring of other parameters (electrolytes, complete blood count, serum biochemistry profile) also may be warranted.

PN Solutions

Basic PN is composed of a protein source (amino acid solutions), a carbohydrate source (dextrose), and a fat source (lipid emulsion). Vitamins, electrolytes, and trace minerals also can be added so that the resulting solution is complete and balanced, at least according to standards for healthy dogs and cats.

PN solutions are mixed in a specific order and under aseptic conditions. Solutions should be made fresh daily, although if properly prepared, they will be stable under refrigeration. Amino acid and dextrose solutions are mixed first, then electrolyte and mineral solutions are added. Great care must be taken when adding combinations of electrolytes, especially phosphorus and calcium, because precipitates can easily form. Next, multivitamins are added, and finally the lipid emulsion. The lipid emulsion is also fragile and the suspended triglyceride particles can coalesce and precipitate. Precipitation of lipid emulsions, or "oiling out," can be detected by visual inspection. There should not be any indication of separation or layering of the final solution. Some recommend delivering PN solutions through a 1.2-micron air-eliminating filter to avoid the potential of lipid embolization.

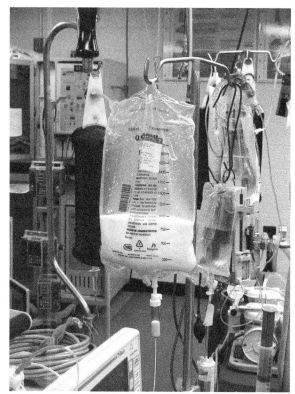

Fig. 2.46. A bag of maintenance crystalloid fluids compounded with a carbohydrate, amino acid, and lipid mixture for parenteral nutrition for a canine patient. The fluid is opaque and yellow from the addition of lipid and a multivitamin. The fluid is homogenous with no evidence of layering or precipitation.

REFERENCES

Armstrong PJ, Hand MS, Frederick GS. Enteral nutrition by tube. *Vet Clin North America Small Anim Pract* 20(1):237–275, 1990.

Bartges J. Symposium on placing feeding tubes. *Vet Med* 99(7):587, 2004.

Bexfield N, Watson P. How to place an oesophagostomy tube. *J Small Anim Pract* 51(2):12–6, 2010.

Bosworth C, Bartges J, Snow P. Nasoesophageal and nasogastric feedings tubes. *Vet Med* 99(7):590–594, 2004.

Crowe DT, Devey JJ. Clinical experience with jejunostomy feeding tubes in 47 small animal patients. *J Vet Emerg Crit Care* 7(1):7–19, 1997.

Crowe DT, Devey JJ. Esophagostomy tubes for feeding and decompression: clinical experiences in 29 small animal patients. *J Am Anim Hosp Assoc* 33:393–403, 1997.

Devitt CM, Seim HB. Clinical evaluation of tube esophagostomy in small animals. *J Amer Anim Hosp Assoc* 33:55–60, 1997.

Eirmann L, Michel KE. Enteral nutrition. In: Silverstein DC, Hopper K (Eds): *Small Animal Critical Care Medicine*. St. Louis: Saunders-Elsevier. pp. 53–58, 2009.

Formaggini L. Normograde, minimally invasive technique for oesophagostomy in cats. *J Fel Med Surg* 11(6):481–486, 2009.

Marks SL. The principles and practical application of enteral nutrition. *Vet Clin North America Small Animal* 28(3):677–708, 1998.

Mazzaferro EM. Esophagostomy tubes: don't underutilize them! *J Vet Emerg Crit Care* 11:153–156, 2001.

McCrackin MA, DeNovo RC, Bright RM, et al: Endoscopic placement of a percutaneous gastroduodenostomy feeding tube in dogs. *J Am Vet Med Assoc* 203:792–797, 1993.

Remillard RL, Armstrong PJ, Davenport DJ. Assisted feeding in hospitalized patients: Enteral and parenteral nutrition. In: Hand MS, Thatcher CD, Remillard RL, Roudebush P. (Eds): *Small Animal Clinical Nutrition 4th Edition*. Topeka, KS: Mark Morris Institute. pp. 351–399.

Swann HM, Sweet DC, Michel K. Complications associated with use of jejunostomy tubes in dogs and cats: 40 cases (1989–1994). *J Am Vet Med Assoc* 210(12):1764–1767, 1997.

Vanatta M, Bartges J, Snow P. Esophagostomy feeding tubes. *Vet Med* 99(7):596–600, 2004.

Waddell LS, Michel KE. Critical care nutrition: Routes of feeding. *Clin Techniques in Sm Anim Pract* 13(4):197–203, 1998.

Wortinger A. Care and use of feeding tubes in dogs and cats. *J Amer Anim Hosp Assoc* 42(5):401–406, 2006.

Thoracocentesis and Thoracostomy Tube Placement

THORACOCENTESIS

Introduction

Thoracocentesis can be both diagnostic and therapeutic in patients with pneumothorax or pleural effusion with respiratory distress. Thoracocentesis should be considered in any patient with respiratory distress and a short, choppy restrictive respiratory pattern caused by pleural effusion or pneumothorax. Thoracic auscultation usually reveals dull muffled heart and lung sounds when intrathoracic, extrapulmonary fluid is present. Other causes of a restrictive respiratory pattern such as pain from fractured ribs, flail chest, pulmonary contusions, pulmonary edema, and lower airway disease should be considered prior to thoracocentesis, or if thoracocentesis is unrewarding.

Supplies Needed

20- to 22-gauge, 1-inch needles
Three-way stop-cock
IV extension tubing
60-ml syringe
Clippers and blades
Nonsterile gloves
Aseptic scrub
Collection basin for fluid
EDTA and red-topped tubes
Sterile culturettes
Port-A-Cul™ for bacterial culture

Veterinary Emergency and Critical Care Procedures, Second Edition. Timothy B. Hackett and Elisa M. Mazzaferro.

Indications

Diagnosis and treatment of:
Pleural effusion
  Hemothorax
  Chylothorax
  Pyothorax
  Neoplastic effusion
  Right-sided cardiac failure
Pneumothorax

Cautions and Contraindications

Caution must be exercised when draining chronic pleural effusions because fibrinous adhesions of the lung to the pleura can occur. In such cases, fluid may be pocketed and difficult to obtain without the use of an ultrasound, and iatrogenic pulmonary puncture could occur.

 | Video available online

Go to www.wiley.com/go/hackett to view a video of this procedure.

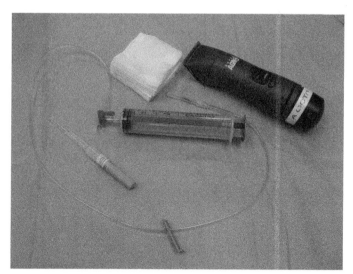

Fig. 3.1. Supplies needed to perform a thoracocentesis include electric clipper and blades; antimicrobial scrub solution; 20- to 22-gauge, 1-inch needles; length of IV extension tubing; three-way stop-cock; 60-ml syringe; red- and lavender-topped tubes for sample analysis; Port-A-Cul™ and sterile culturettes for bacterial culture; and a collection basin for fluid.

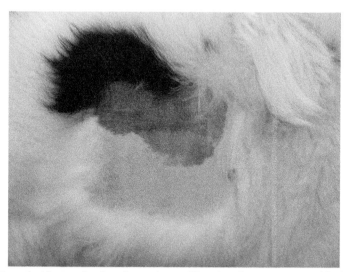

Fig. 3.2. Place the patient in sternal or lateral recumbency. Clip a 4- to 8-cm square area of fur in the middle of the chest.

Helpful hint: It is best to perform the thoracocentesis between the seventh and tenth intercostal space. Visualize the entire lateral thoracic wall as a box, and clip a square in the center of a box. This helps save valuable time that is often spent counting rib spaces when performing an emergency thoracocentesis.

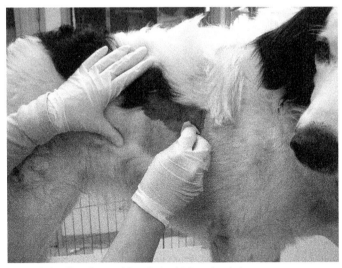

Fig. 3.3. Aseptically scrub the clipped area with antimicrobial scrub solution.

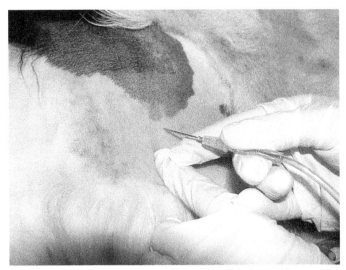

Fig. 3.4. Palpate the rib spaces in the middle of the box. The needle will be inserted between ribs, avoiding the caudal aspect of each rib, where the intercostal arteries lie.

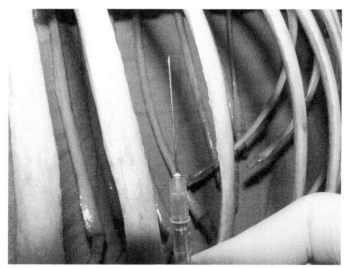

Fig. 3.5. Find the bevel of the needle. Mark the hub of the needle or the extension tubing in line with the bevel. This will allow the bevel of the needle to be rotated toward the center of the patient as the needle is inserted through the skin, perpendicular to the body wall.

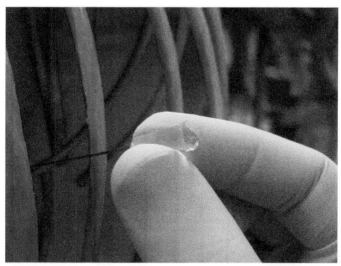

Fig. 3.6. Insert the needle in between rib spaces in the center of the clipped area. Alternatively, place a drop of sterile water or sterile 0.9% saline in the hub of the needle, and insert the needle perpendicularly between rib spaces. Once the needle is in the pleural space, the hanging drop of saline or water will be sucked into the needle and pleural cavity.

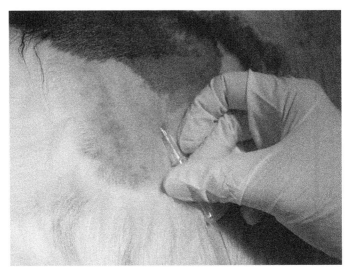

Fig. 3.7. Once you are in the pleural space, direct the needle parallel with the body wall to avoid iatrogenic lung puncture. The needle can be pivoted like the hands of a clock, such that the needle always stays parallel with the body wall. The bevel of the needle should be directed dorsally to obtain air, and ventrally to obtain fluid.

Helpful hint: You may insert the needle directly into the epaxial muscles if you attempt to insert the needle too far dorsally on the chest wall. Inserting the needle in the center of the box, then sweeping the bevel of the needle dorsally, will increase your chances of a positive tap in cases of pneumothorax. Attach the male port of the length of IV extension tubing to the hub of the needle. Never let go of the needle.

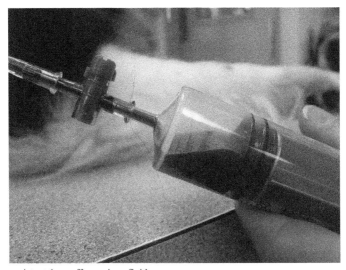

Fig. 3.8. Have an assistant draw off any air or fluid.

Helpful hint: Remember to quantify the volume air or fluid you are obtaining from each side. Remove the needle when you obtain negative pressure. No bandage is necessary. Thoracocentesis is usually performed on both sides of the chest because the mediastinum doesn't always communicate. Placement of a thoracostomy tube is indicated if negative pressure cannot be obtained or maintained in cases of pneumothorax.

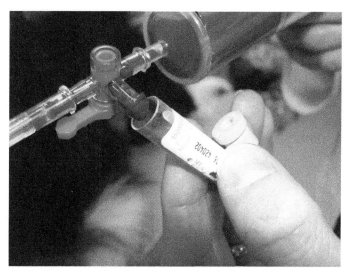

Fig. 3.9. Save any fluid collected in sterile red- and lavender topped collection tubes for later culture and fluid analysis.

THORACOSTOMY TUBE PLACEMENT

Introduction

Placement of a thoracostomy tube can be life-saving in cases of tension pneumothorax or recurrent simple pneumothorax. Once a thoracostomy tube has been placed, it can be connected to a suction apparatus that continuously drains free air from within the pleural space until primary lung pathology has had time to heal. Hypoxemia is treated or prevented by allowing the lungs to remain expanded.

In other cases, the tube can be used to infuse and evacuate sterile saline from the thoracic cavity during the medical management of pyothorax. A small amount of fluid will develop simply because of the presence of the tube within the pleural cavity. Tubes can be removed if air production has ceased for 24 hours. Cytology is used to determine the ongoing need for thoracic drainage when treating inflammatory pleural effusion. White blood cell count and morphology, along with the absence of bacteria, are useful indices for tube removal.

Supplies Needed

Sterile gloves
Electric clippers and blades
Antimicrobial scrub solution
2% lidocaine with 24-gauge needle
3- to 6-ml syringe
Sterile surgical pack
   Sterile field towels (4)
   Towel clamps
   Number 10 scalpel blade
   Scalpel handle
Needle holders
Mayo scissors
Thumb forceps
Hemostats
Gauze, 4-inch × 4-inch squares
Argyle thoracic drainage tube with trocar stylette
Sterile drapes
3–0 or 2–0 nonabsorbable suture
1-inch tape
Christmas tree adapter
3-way stop-cock
IV extension tubing
Wire
Wire cutters
Antimicrobial ointment

Indications

Pneumothorax
  Continuous suction
  Intermittent suction
Pleural effusion
Pleural lavage for medical management of pyothorax

Contraindications

Coagulopathies
Pleural adhesions

 Video available online

Go to www.wiley.com/go/hackett to view a video of this procedure.

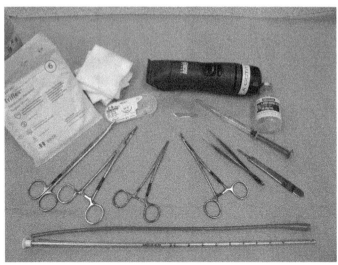

Fig. 3.10. Supplies needed for thoracostomy tube placement include sterile gloves, antimicrobial scrub, 2% lidocaine, sterile needle and syringe, surgical instruments, Argyle thoracic drain with trocar, suture, Christmas tree adapter, three-way stop-cock, IV extension tubing, surgical wire, wire cutters, antimicrobial ointment, and bandaging material.

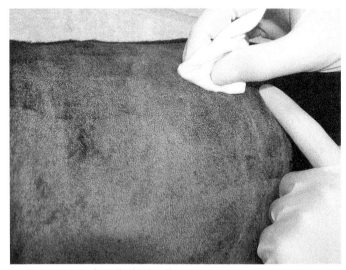

Fig. 3.11. Clip the entire lateral thoracic wall with the clipper blades, and then aseptically scrub the clipped area.

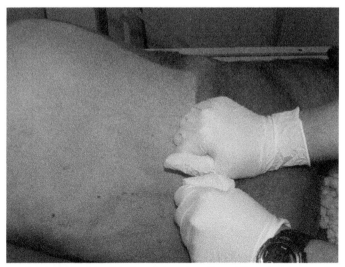

Fig. 3.12. Have an assistant pull the skin of the lateral thoracic wall cranially and ventrally at the point of the elbow.

> **Helpful hint:** This will help to create a subcutaneous tunnel through which the thoracostomy tube will pass.

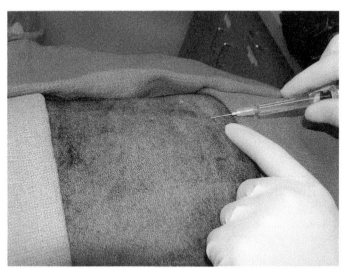

Fig. 3.13. Insert 1 mg/kg 2% lidocaine from the tenth to seventh intercostal space. Make sure the block includes the intercostal muscles through which the tube and trocar will pass.

> **Helpful hint:** Leave the needle in the skin to indicate where the lidocaine was placed.

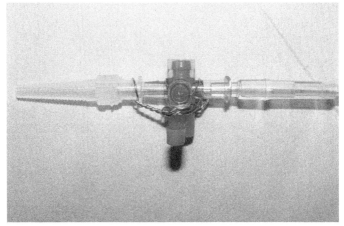

Fig. 3.14. While the lidocaine is taking effect, prepare the thoracostomy tube and assemble the IV extension tubing, three-way stop-cock, Christmas tree adapter, and 60-ml syringe. Secure the three-way stop-cock, Christmas tree adapter to the tube with orthopedic wire.

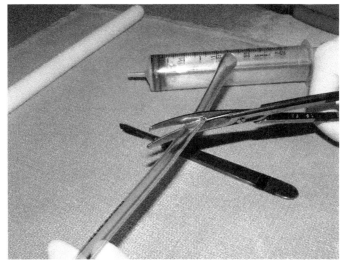

Fig. 3.15. Remove the trocar from the thoracic tube and cut the proximal tip of the tube on a diagonal so that the Christmas tree adapter will fit securely in the opening.

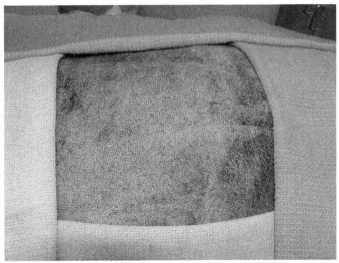

Fig. 3.16. Drape the lateral thorax with sterile field towels secured with towel clamps.

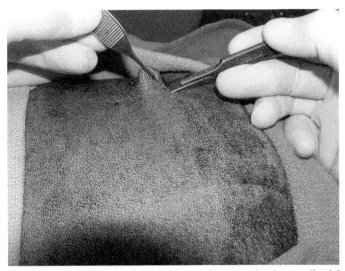

Fig. 3.17. Tent the skin at the dorsal portion of the tenth intercostal space, and make a small stab incision through the skin, making the hole just large enough for the tube to pass.

Helpful hint: If the incision is too large, air can leak around the tube such that suction may not be efficient.

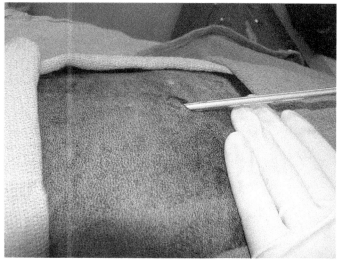

Fig. 3.18. Insert the trocar back into the thoracostomy tube. Insert the trocar and tube through the skin incision, tunneling the apparatus cranially.

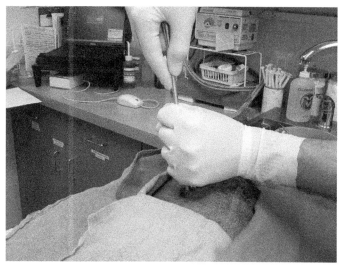

Fig. 3.19. When the tip of the trocar is over the seventh intercostal space, direct the trocar perpendicular to the thoracic wall. Grasp the trocar at the level of the skin firmly, and using the palm of your hand, push the trocar through the intercostal space into the thorax.

Helpful hint: Stand on a stool or lower the table to increase your leverage and make this step easier for you and the patient.

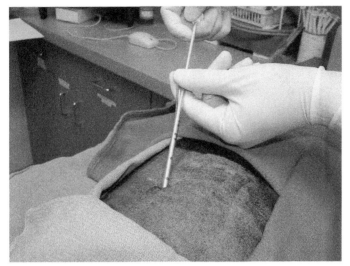

Fig. 3.20. Once the trocar has entered the thorax, push the tube off of the trocar cranially and ventrally, and have the assistant release the skin.

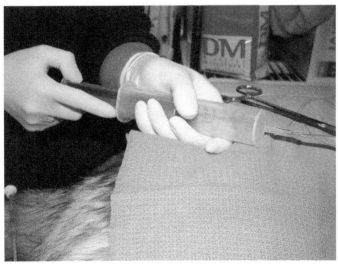

Fig. 3.21. Immediately secure the Christmas-tree adapter set-up, and have an assistant evacuate the thorax while you are securing the tube.

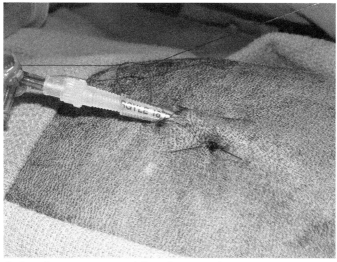

Fig. 3.22. Place a horizontal mattress suture cranially to the purse-string suture, around the tube. Use care to not puncture the tube, and don't make the suture so tight to occlude blood flow and cause skin damage.

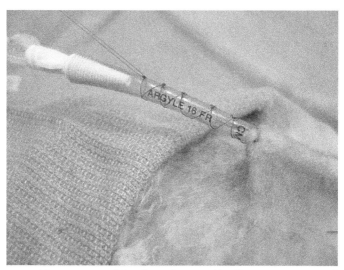

Fig. 3.23. Place a purse-string suture around the tube, and secure with a finger-trap to prevent tube displacement caudally. To protect the tube site from contamination, place a piece of 4-inch × 4-inch gauze with antimicrobial ointment over the chest tube point of entry into the skin, and secure to the thorax with layers of roll gauze, Kling®, and Elasticon®.

Helpful hint: Make sure that some of the adhesive tape is attached to the fur at the cranial edge of the bandage, to ensure that the bandage does not slip caudally.

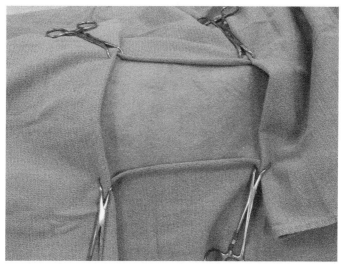

Fig. 3.24. Clip, aseptically scrub, then drape the lateral thorax as previously described.

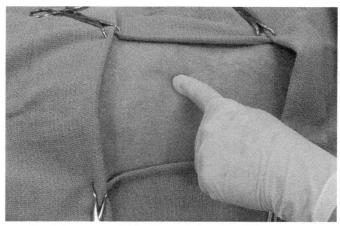

Fig. 3.25. Palpate the seventh to ninth intercostal space.

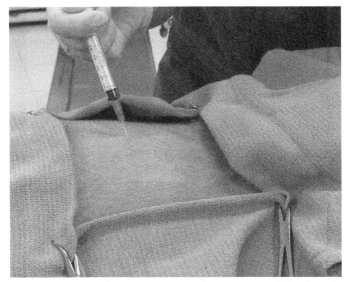

Fig. 3.26. Insert lidocaine through the skin and intercostal muscles at the proposed site of tube insertion. During this time, have an assistant pull the skin of the lateral thorax cranially toward the elbow.

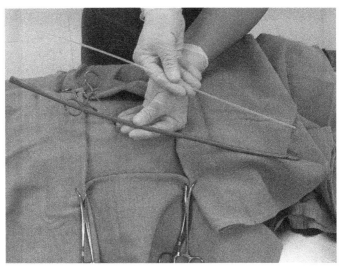

Fig. 3.27. Measure the red rubber catheter from the tube entrance site to the fifth intercostal space. A polypropylene rigid catheter that is smaller in diameter than the red rubber catheter can be inserted into the red rubber catheter to make the device more rigid during insertion.

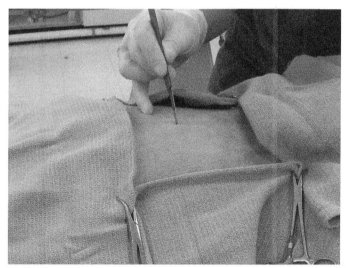

Fig. 3.28. Make an incision through the skin at the seventh to ninth intercostal space.

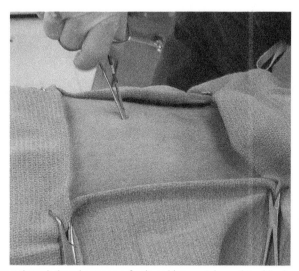

Fig. 3.29. Bluntly dissect through the subcutaneous fascia and intercostal muscles with a hemostat forceps. Bluntly pop through the intercostal muscles into the pleural space.

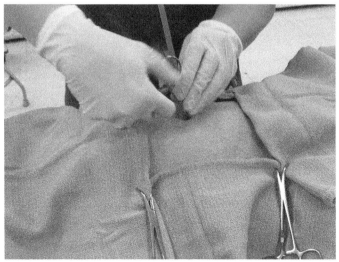

Fig. 3.30. Insert the red rubber catheter and its polypropylene stylette through the open tips of the hemostat and into the pleural cavity, and direct it cranioventrally so that the tip is at approximately the fifth intercostal space.

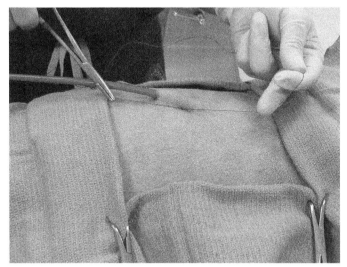

Fig. 3.31. Place a horizontal mattress suture under the tube just caudal to the point the tube enters the thoracic wall. This will pull skin and subcutaneous tissues around the tube, preventing air or fluid in the thorax from accumulating under the skin.

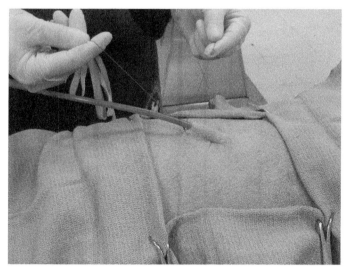
Fig. 3.32. Place a series of finger-trap sutures around the tube to secure it in place, then bandage.

MANAGEMENT OF AN OPEN SUCKING CHEST WOUND

Introduction

Open sucking chest wounds secondary to blunt or penetrating thoracic trauma are a life-threatening emergency that must be treated immediately. Pneumothorax and secondary hypoxemia cannot resolve without restoring negative intrapleural pressure. This requires a tight seal over the wound preventing communication of atmospheric air with the pleural space. Once the chest wound has been sealed, thoracocentesis and thoracostomy tube placement can be performed to allow expansion of the lungs until definitive wound repair can be accomplished.

Supplies Needed

Electric clippers and blades
Sterile lubricating jelly or antimicrobial ointment
Sterile surgical gloves
Sterile scissors
Cotton roll gauze
Kling® or brown gauze
Elasticon® or Vetrap™

Indications

Penetrating or blunt trauma with open communication through the wound into the thorax

Contraindications

Tension pneumothorax

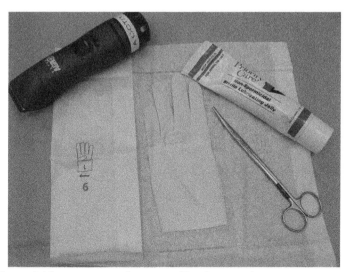

Fig. 3.33. Supplies needed for management of an open sucking chest wound.

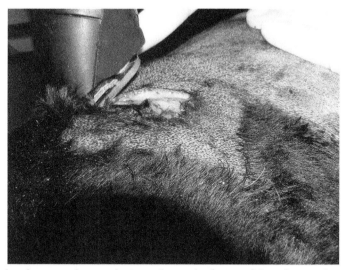

Fig. 3.34. Clip a broad area over the open chest wound, removing fur around the entire wound.

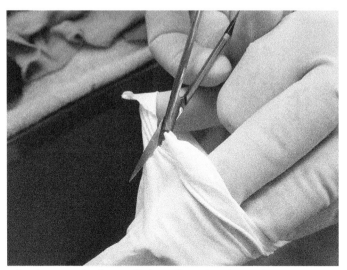

Fig. 3.35. With sterile scissors, cut the fingers off of a sterile surgical glove and cut open the glove to create a flat sterile latex patch. Alternatively, surgical sticky drape can be used to achieve the same result.

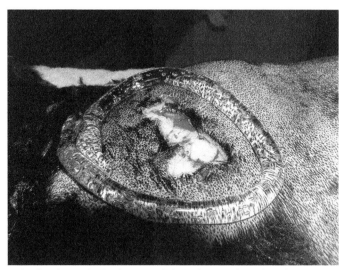

Fig. 3.36. Place a strip of sterile lubricating jelly or antibiotic ointment circumferentially around the chest wound.

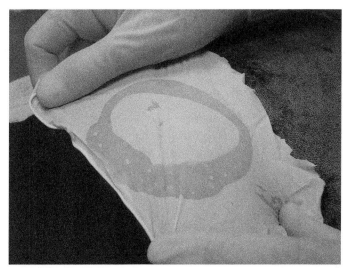

Fig. 3.37. Place the sterile glove over the wound, making sure that the glove is in contact with and covers the lubricating jelly to create a seal. After creating a seal, a thoracic drain can be placed as previously described. Take care to NOT place the tube through the wound. The thoracic drain should stay in place until definitive surgical exploration and repair of the chest wound can occur once the patient is more stable.

LOCAL ANESTHETIC BLOCKS FOR RIB FRACTURES OR FLAIL CHEST

Introduction

The pain associated with rib fractures impairs a patient's ability to adequately ventilate and thus move oxygen into the lungs. Hypoxemia from blunt thoracic trauma, pneumothorax, and underlying pulmonary contusions is exacerbated by impaired ventilatory capacity. Rather than wrapping rib fractures, which causes further restriction to thoracic excursions, applying local anesthesia to the nerves supplying affected ribs can greatly improve ventilatory function.

Supplies Needed

3- to 6-ml syringe
22-gauge, 3/4-inch and 1–1/2-inch needles
Lidocaine 2%
Sodium bicarbonate
Electric clippers and blades
Antimicrobial scrub

Indications

Rib fractures

Contraindications

Known sensitivity to local anesthetic agents

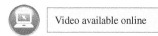 Video available online

Go to www.wiley.com/go/hackett to view a video of this procedure.

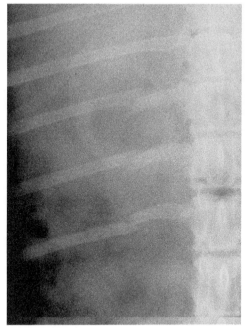

Fig. 3.38. Thoracic radiograph with rib fractures.

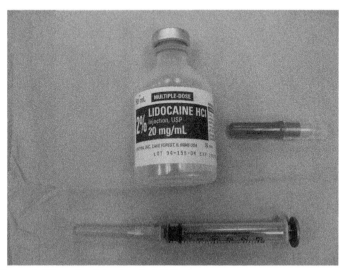

Fig. 3.39. Supplies needed for analgesic treatment of rib fractures.

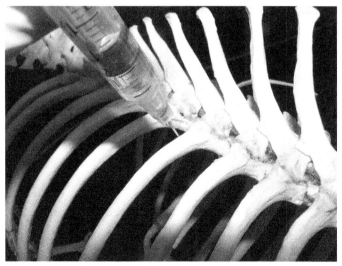

Fig. 3.40. Skeleton and placement of local anesthetic blocks. The local anesthetic will be placed at the dorsal and caudal aspect of each rib.

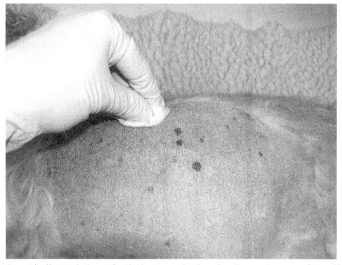

Fig. 3.41. Clip and aseptically scrub the patient's thorax on the dorsal and ventral aspect of the affected ribs, making sure that the rib cranial and caudal to the affected rib(s) is included.

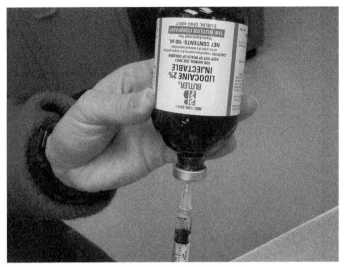

Fig. 3.42. Draw up 1 mg/kg of 2% lidocaine.

Helpful hint: Add a small amount of sodium bicarbonate (1:9 ratio of bicarbonate to lidocaine) to decrease the pain associated with infusion of this acidic solution. It was previously thought that sodium bicarbonate decreased the efficacy of lidocaine. However, recent evidence has demonstrated that the two can be mixed without decreasing the efficacy of this acidic local anesthetic. Warming the lidocaine to body temperature and infusing SLOWLY also aids in decreasing patient discomfort.

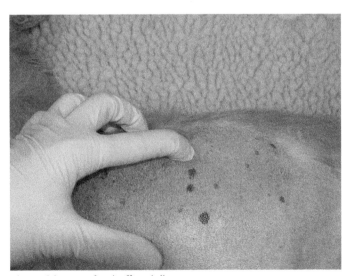

Fig. 3.43. Palpate the caudal aspect of each affected rib.

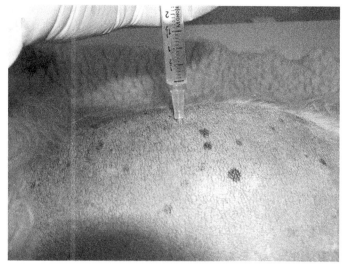

Fig. 3.44. Infuse a small amount of the lidocaine/bicarbonate mixture at the dorsal-caudal and ventrocaudal aspect of each rib. Repeat the process for each affected rib and at least one rib cranial and one rib caudal to the affected rib(s) segment. This process can be repeated up to three times daily, as needed, for adjunctive analgesia.

Helpful hint: Always aspirate prior to injecting, to avoid intravenous injection.

REFERENCES

Aron DN, Roberts RE. Pneumothorax. In: Bojrab NJ (Ed): *Disease Mechanisms in Small Animal Surgery*. Philadelphia: Lea & Febiger, p. 396, 1993.

MacPhail C. Thoracic Injuries. In: Wingfield WE, Raffee M (Eds): *The Veterinary ICU Book*. Jackson, WY: Teton NewMedia, pp. 655–669, 2002.

Mazzaferro EM. Respiratory injury. In: Wingfield WE, Raffee M (Eds): *The Veterinary ICU Book*. Jackson, WY: Teton NewMedia, pp. 935–956, 2002.

Taylor NS. Thoracic drainage. In: Wingfield WE (Ed): *Veterinary Emergency Secrets 2nd Edition*. Philadelphia: Hanley and Belfus, p. 436, 2002.

CHAPTER 4

Oxygen Supplementation and Respiratory Sampling Techniques

NASAL AND NASOPHARYNGEAL OXYGEN CATHETER PLACEMENT

Introduction

The placement of a nasal or nasopharyngeal tube is a quick and simple means to provide supplemental oxygen to the hypoxic patient. Nasal and nasopharyngeal oxygen catheters are well-tolerated, require minimal equipment, and are easy to maintain.

Supplies Needed

Argyle feeding tube or red rubber catheter
3–0 nylon suture
Surgical staples
2% lidocaine or 0.5% proparacaine
Permanent marker
Sterile lubricating gel or ointment
1-ml syringe case
Flexible extension tubing
Humidified oxygen source
Rigid Elizabethan collar

Indications

Hypoxemia due to any cause

Veterinary Emergency and Critical Care Procedures, Second Edition. Timothy B. Hackett and Elisa M. Mazzaferro.
© 2012 John Wiley & Sons, Inc. Published 2012 by John Wiley & Sons, Inc.

Contraindications

Laryngeal obstruction
Nasal or facial trauma
Epistaxis
Coagulopathies
Nasal mass lesions
   Neoplasia
   Foreign bodies
   Fungal infection
Relatively contraindicated in patients with intracranial mass lesions or elevated intracranial
    pressure due to the risk of sneezing and increasing intracranial pressure during catheter
    placement

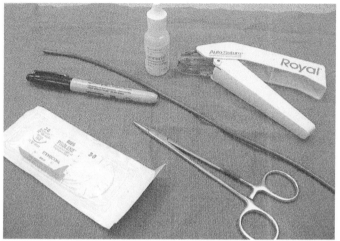

Fig. 4.1. Supplies needed for placement of a nasal or nasopharyngeal oxygen supplementation tube.

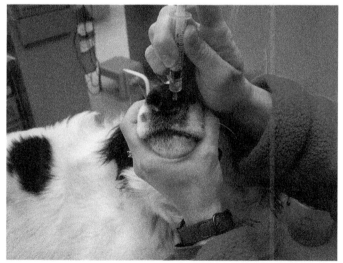

Fig. 4.2. Instill several drops of dilute 2% lidocaine or proparacaine in the nostril, tilting the patient's nose upward to assure coating of the nasal mucosa with the topical anesthetic.

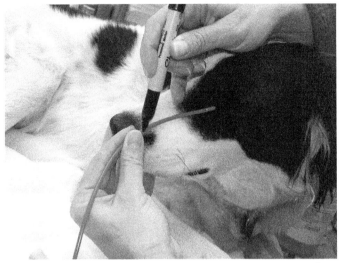

Fig. 4.3. For placement of a nasal oxygen catheter, the tip of the tube is placed to the level of the lateral canthus of the eye, and the portion adjacent to the tip of the nose marked with a permanent marker.

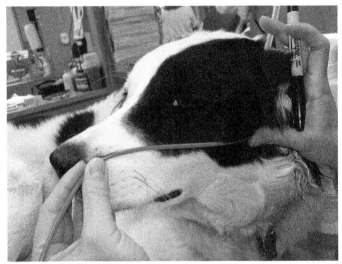

Fig. 4.4. For placement of a nasopharyngeal oxygen catheter, the tip of the tube is measured from the ramus of the mandible to the tip of the nose, and marked accordingly.

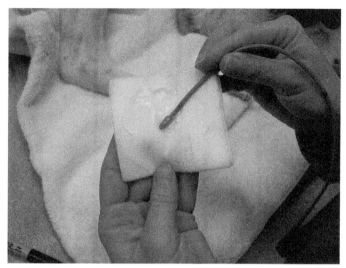

Fig. 4.5. Lubricate the tip of the tube with sterile lubricant jelly or ointment.

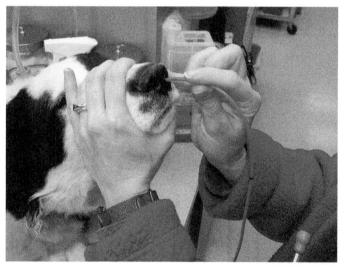

Fig. 4.6. Hold the tube as close to the tip as possible, adjacent and as close to the nostril as possible. Hold the patient's muzzle with the other hand while an assistant restrains the patient. Direct the tube ventrally and medially into the nostril to the level of the mark on the tube.

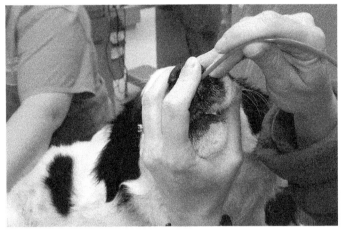

Fig. 4.7. When placing a nasopharyngeal oxygen catheter, pinch the dorsolateral portion of the external nares medially, and push the nasal philtrum dorsally as you attempt to pass the tube into the nasopharynx. This maneuver will help facilitate passing the tube into the ventral nasal meatus, then into the nasopharynx.

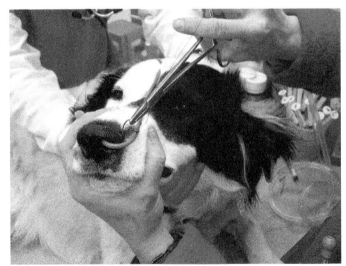

Fig. 4.8. Place a stay suture adjacent to the nostril, then secure the tube to the stay suture with another length of suture. If the tube becomes dislodged, the stay suture can remain in place, avoiding this somewhat uncomfortable step when you replace the tube.

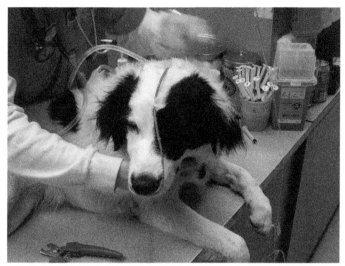

Fig. 4.9. Suture the tube to the stay suture with a finger-trap. Place a second and third suture either over the dorsal nasal planum and on top of the head, or on the lateral maxilla and zygomatic arch. Immediately place a rigid Elizabethan collar to avoid patient disruption or removal of the tube. Oxygen flow rates of 50 ml to 100 ml/kg/ minute are well-tolerated, provided that the oxygen source is humidified to prevent drying of the nasal mucosa. Topical proparacaine (0.5%) can be instilled as necessary for patient comfort.

Helpful hint: Avoid the whiskers when suturing, because trapping them in the suture and tube can cause patient discomfort.

OXYGEN HOOD

Introduction

Oxygen hoods are an excellent method of providing short-term supplemental oxygen support to the hypoxemic patient. Hoods are available commercially, or can be manufactured using a rigid Elizabethan collar, plastic wrap, and adhesive tape. In some cases, patients will not tolerate an oxygen hood. Also, the patient can become hyperthermic and must be monitored closely to prevent hyperthermia from occurring. Extremely small patients can be placed directly into a hood for supplemental oxygen without the stress of any handling.

Supplies Needed

Commercially available oxygen hood
Rigid Elizabethan collar
Plastic wrap
White adhesive tape
Flexible oxygen tubing
Humidified oxygen source

Indications

Hypoxemia due to any cause

Contraindications

Anxiety and intolerance of the hood
Panting
Hyperthermia

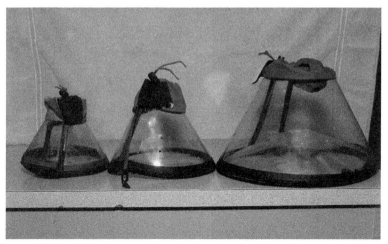

Fig. 4.10. Commercially available oxygen hoods.

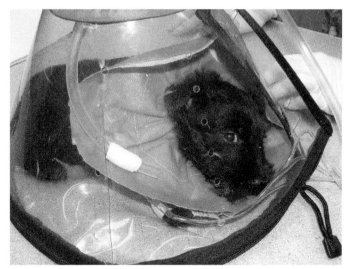

Fig. 4.11. In some cases, a small puppy, kitten, or exotic species can be fit into an oxygen hood to create a small oxygen cage.

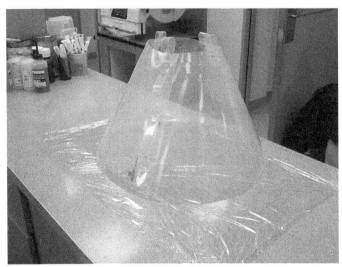

Fig. 4.12. To manufacture your own oxygen hood, cover the front three-fourths of a rigid Elizabethan collar with plastic wrap.

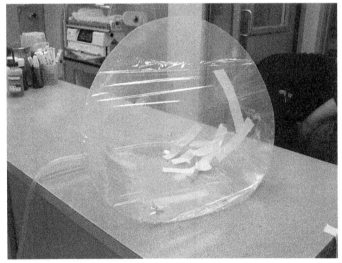

Fig. 4.13. Secure the plastic wrap in place with white adhesive tape.

Helpful hint: Leave the bottom fourth of the hood open to prevent iatrogenic hyperthermia and condensation.

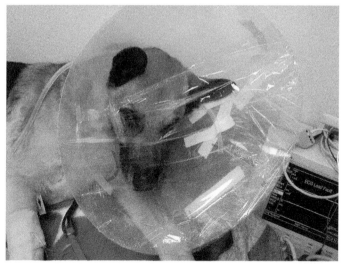

Fig. 4.14. Secure the hood around the patient's head with a length of gauze. Insert a length of flexible oxygen tubing into the side of the hood and administer supplemental oxygen at 50 ml to 100 ml/kg/minute.

INTRATRACHEAL OXYGEN SUPPLEMENTATION CATHETER

Introduction

The placement of an intratracheal catheter for oxygen supplementation is an effective and well-tolerated means of providing supplemental oxygen to the patient with head trauma, nasopharyngeal obstruction, pulmonary parenchymal disease, and hypoventilation. Placement may require sedation or general anesthesia in some patients.

Supplies Needed

Cook Surgi-VET chest drainage tube OR Venocath®16-gauge over-the-wire long catheter
Electric clippers and blades
Heavy sedation or general anesthesia protocol
Antimicrobial scrub
Number 10 and number 11 scalpel blade on scalpel handle
Small Gelpi retractors (2)
Curved mosquito hemostats
Mayo or Mettzenbaum scissors
Groove director from spay pack
3–0 nylon suture
1-inch white tape
Cotton bandage material
Roll gauze
ElastiKon® or Vetrap™
1-ml syringe case
Flexible oxygen tubing
Humidified oxygen source
Sterile gloves
Sterile field towels (4)
Backhaus towel clamps (4)

Indications

Refractory hypoxemia with nasal or nasopharyngeal oxygen supplementation
Patient will not tolerate nasal or nasopharyngeal oxygen catheter
Head or facial trauma
Nasal trauma
Epistaxis
Coagulopathies
Nasal obstruction
    Trauma
    Mass lesion
Refractory hypoxemia in patients in which mechanical ventilation is not possible

Contraindications

Tracheal injury
Tracheal obstruction distal to site of catheter placement

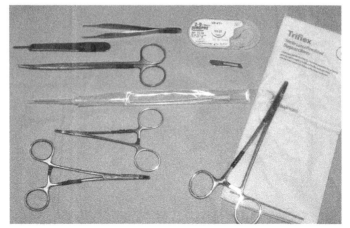

Fig. 4.15. Supplies needed for intratracheal oxygen catheter.

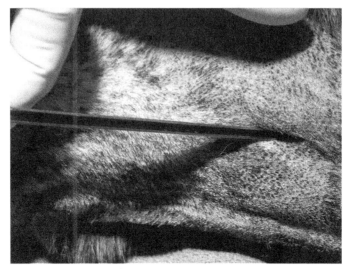

Fig. 4.16. Insert a grooved director into the incision, and then remove the hemostat.

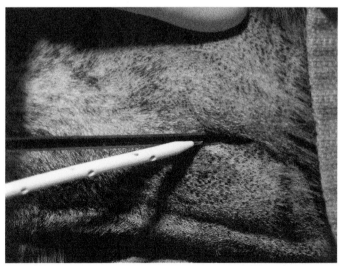

Fig. 4.17. Insert the Cook Surgi-VET chest drainage tube or Venocath®16-gauge over-the-wire long catheter into the lumen of the trachea. Once the catheter is inserted about halfway, remove the trocar, and continue inserting the catheter such that the distal end of the catheter is situated at the level of the carina. In large dogs, the catheter may be inserted to its hub.

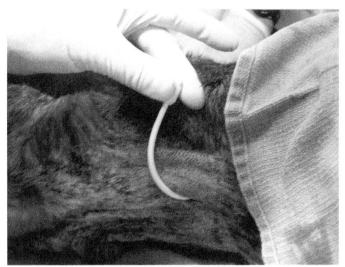

Fig. 4.18. Secure the catheter to the skin with a length of 3–0 nylon suture to a length of white tape secured around the catheter. Place a piece of 1-inch white tape around the catheter and secure it to the neck. Loosely bandage the catheter to the neck, then secure the syringe adapter and appropriate length of oxygen tubing and connect both to a humidified oxygen source.

Helpful hint: Make sure that the catheter can move freely with minimal resistance to prevent kinking of the catheter at the point of insertion into the neck.

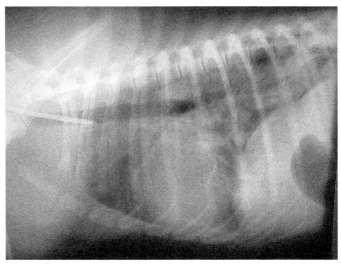

Fig. 4.19. Lateral thoracic radiograph of intratracheal oxygen catheter in place in a patient with acute respiratory distress syndrome (ARDS).

TRACHEOSTOMY TUBE PLACEMENT

Introduction and Indications

A temporary tracheostomy tube should be placed in cases of severe upper airway obstruction, trauma, or laryngeal or pharyngeal collapse, or if long-term positive pressure ventilation will be performed.

Supplies Needed

Sterile field towels (4)
Backhaus towel clamps (4)
Number 10 and number 11 scalpel blades
Scalpel handle
Small Gelpi retractors (2)
Sterile Mettzenbaum scissors
Curved Kelly hemostats (1)
Gauze, 4-inch × 4-inch squares
3–0 to 2–0 nylon suture
Various sized Shiley tracheostomy tubes
Umbilical tape
Electric clippers and blades
Antimicrobial scrub
Sterile gloves

Contraindications

Tracheal injury
Tracheal obstruction distal to tracheostomy site

Note: The initial management and preparation of a patient for placement of an intratracheal oxygen catheter is identical for the placement of a tracheostomy tube. Please refer to the tracheostomy tube section for photos and a general overview of the technique unless indicated.

(1) Heavily sedate the patient or place the patient under general anesthesia. Place the patient in dorsal recumbency.

> **Helpful hint:** It is useful to place the patient in a V-trough to ensure that the patient is in the correct position. This is helpful to assist you in making sure to stay on the ventral midline.

(2) Clip the ventral cervical region from the ramus of the mandible caudally to the thoracic inlet and dorsally to the epaxial muscles.

> **Helpful hint:** In patients with long fur, clip the long feathers short to ensure and maintain sterility of the surgical field.

(3) Aseptically scrub the clipped area and drape the area with sterile field towels secured with Backhaus towel clamps.

(4) Palpate the larynx. Make a 1-cm skin incision perpendicular to the trachea with a number 10 scalpel blade, just caudal to the larynx.

> **Helpful hint:** Make sure that you stay on ventral midline.

(5) Bluntly dissect through the underlying fascia with a curved hemostats or Mettzenbaum scissors to the level of the trachea.

> **Helpful hint:** Make sure that you dissect only in the same plane to prevent traumatic injury to the sternohyoid muscles and help facilitate exposure of the underlying trachea.

(6) Retract the skin and underlying musculature with a Gelpi retractors to improve exposure and visualization of the trachea.

(7) Visualize the trachea. Gently pick up the overlying fascia and snip with a Mettzenbaum scissors to expose tracheal rings.

> **Helpful hint:** Make sure that you avoid any vessels, because hemorrhage will obscure visibility in the surgical field.

(8) Make a small stab incision with a number 11 scalpel blade between tracheal rings.

> **Helpful hint:** Only a small incision is necessary. DO NOT incise more than 50% of the circumference of the trachea. Insert the tips of a curved hemostat into the incision.

 Video available online

Go to www.wiley.com/go/hackett to view a video of this procedure.

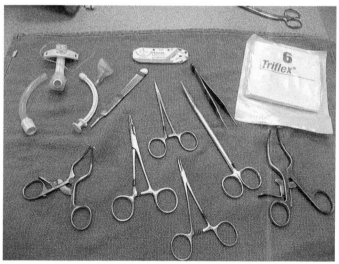

Fig. 4.20. Supplies needed for temporary tracheostomy tube placement.

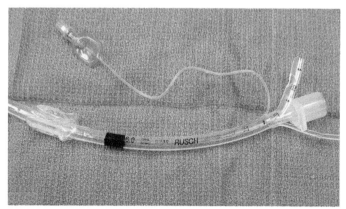

Fig. 4.21. If a Shiley tracheostomy tube is not available, a tracheostomy tube can be made from a low-pressure cuffed endotracheal tube. To create a tracheostomy tube, cut the proximal end of the tube above the tube that inflates the low pressure cuff distally. The tube can be cut such that the proximal end of the tube folds down to create wings that can be secured to the neck with umbilical tape.

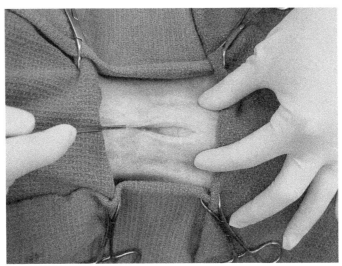

Fig. 4.22. Place the patient under general anesthesia, and then place the patient in dorsal recumbency. Clip and then aseptically scrub the ventral cervical region from the ramus of the mandible caudally to the thoracic inlet and dorsally to midline. Drape the sterile field with sterile towels secured with towel clamps. Next, palpate the larynx, and make a 3- to 6-cm skin incision on the ventral midline, perpendicular to the trachea, using a number 10 scalpel blade.

Helpful hint: It is useful to place the patient in a V-trough to make sure that the patient is in the correct position. This is helpful to assist you in making sure to stay on the ventral midline. Make sure that the head and neck are completely straight.

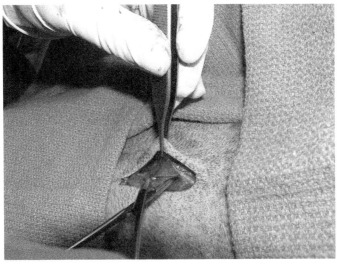

Fig. 4.23. Bluntly dissect the underlying subcutaneous tissue and through the sternohyoideus muscles using a curved hemostats or Mettzenbaum scissors.

Helpful hint: Use care to dissect through the same muscle plane and avoid vessels. This will aid rapid visualization of the trachea and prevent hemorrhage.

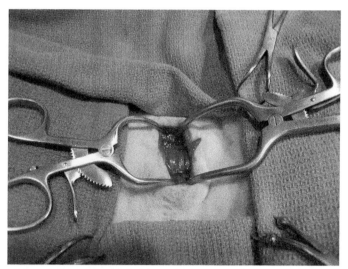

Fig. 4.24. Retract the lateral edges of the skin incision and subcutaneous tissues, including the sternohyoideus muscles, laterally to allow the best visualization.

Helpful hint: The use of Gelpi retractors facilitates a quick dissection.

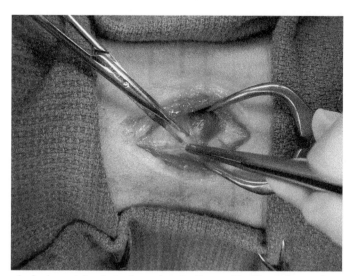

Fig. 4.25. Pick up the fascia overlying the trachea and gently dissect with a Mettzenbaum scissors.

Helpful hint: Use care to avoid vessels to prevent hemorrhage and impaired visualization in your surgical field.

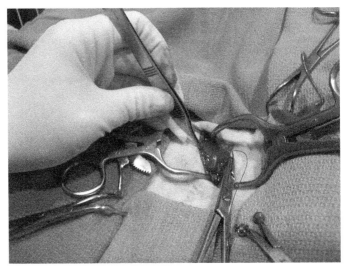

Fig. 4.26. Place two individual stay sutures with 0 or 1 nonabsorbable suture around a tracheal ring just proximal (toward the thoracic inlet) to the incision. Keep the ends of the suture long and keep the ends out of the final bandage. This suture will allow you to exteriorize the trachea, simplifying placement of the tracheostomy tube. This suture remains in place until the patient no longer requires the tracheostomy tube. It will be very important if you need to replace the tube.

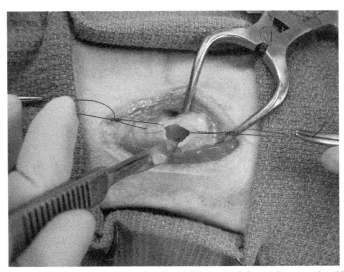

Fig. 4.27. Make a horizontal incision between the fourth and fifth tracheal rings using a number 10 scalpel blade, taking care to avoid cutting more than 50% of the circumference of the trachea.

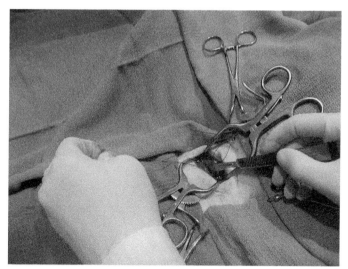

Fig. 4.28. Retract the stay sutures to open the tracheostomy incision, and place a Shiley tracheostomy catheter into the lumen of the trachea.

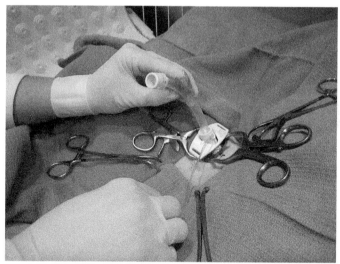

Fig. 4.29. If a Shiley tracheostomy tube is not available, an appropriately sized endotracheal tube can be cut down and splayed open to create a short tube with lateral handles. Care should be taken to preserve the cuff and its inflation tubing.

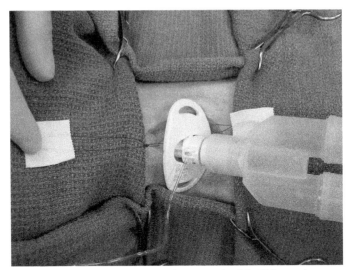

Fig. 4.30. Remove the internal obturator, and secure the inner cannula of the Shiley tracheostomy catheter in place. Next, secure the oxygen source as necessary. Secure the outer cannula to the neck with a length of umbilical tape. The tube can be removed once the patient no longer requires the tracheostomy tube. Next, remove the stay sutures, and leave the wound to heal by second intention.

AIRWAY PRESSURE THERAPY

Introduction

Many causes of acute respiratory distress result in reduced tidal volumes and the collapse of respiratory alveoli. Reduced tidal volumes reduce the compliance of the lungs. A normally compliant lung allows the exchange of gasses with very little energy. Small changes in intrathoracic pressure result in large changes in respiratory volume. As lung volumes are decreased, the energy required for moving fresh air into the lungs increases. Patients have to work much harder to breathe.

Airway pressure therapy allows the clinician to take over much of the work of breathing to allow improved movement of air into and out of the lung. This helps re-expand and recruit collapsed alveoli and bring resting lung volumes back toward normal, making breathing more efficient.

Positive end-expiratory pressure (PEEP) is applied to intubated patients in an effort to maintain resting lung volumes. In patients with reduced resting lung volumes, end-expiratory pressure can maintain inflation so that lungs remain compliant.

Supplies Needed

Anesthetic circuit with a cuffed endotracheal tube
CO_2 scavenging system
Pressure manometer
Oxygen source

Indications

Hypoventilation
Hypoxemia despite supplemental oxygen
 Pulmonary edema
 Pulmonary contusions

Contraindications

Shock: Increased airway pressures can increase intrathoracic pressures. Hypotensive shock patients can see cardiac pre-load reduced with further drops in blood pressure when intrathoracic pressures rise with positive airway pressures.
Diseases with increased pulmonary compliance (e.g., asthma, emphysema)

 Video available online

Go to www.wiley.com/go/hackett to view a video of this procedure.

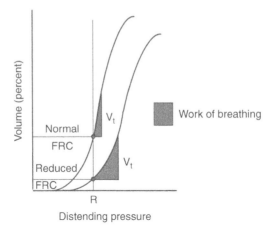

Fig. 4.31. The pressure volume curve showing the relationship between distending pressure and lung volumes. The sigmoid curve on the left represents a normal lung. The functional residual capacity (FRC) is the volume of air remaining in the lung at the end of a normal breath. At this volume it requires a small change in pressure to take a tidal breath (V_t). The curve on the right represents a patient with poor compliance and reduced FRC. This patient needs to expend more energy for the same change in volume.

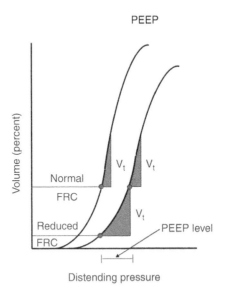

Fig. 4.32. This graph shows what happens to the patient with reduced pulmonary compliance and FRC when positive end-expiratory pressure (PEEP) is applied to the airway. The PEEP maintains a higher FRC. The result is less work required for a normal tidal breath.

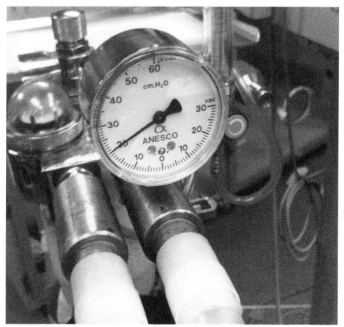

Fig. 4.33. The pressure manometer closest the patient is used to monitor airway pressure therapy. With a cuffed endotracheal tube in place the patient is given a breath to a maximum pressure of 20 cm H_2O.

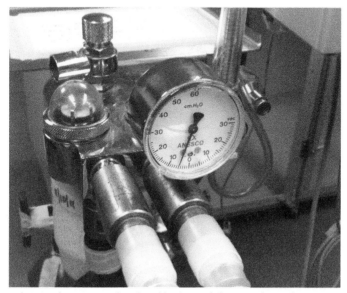

Fig. 4.34. With gentle manual pressure on the rebreathing bag and close attention to the manometer, PEEP is maintained at 5 cm H_2O during exhalation. The manometer is not allowed to fall below the chosen level of PEEP (5 cm H_2O in this example).

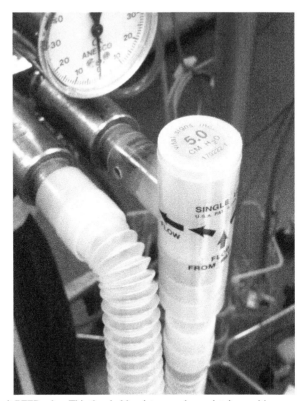

Fig. 4.35. An in-circuit PEEP valve. This threshold resistance valve maintains positive pressure within the airway. This PEEP valve is designed to maintain 5 cm H_2O at the end of expiration.

TRANSORAL WASH

Introduction

A transoral wash may be performed whenever samples of the airway are required for bacterial or viral culture, or to obtain cells for cytologic evaluation. Although brochoalveolar lavage (BAL) is considered to be the gold standard for obtaining airway samples, it requires expensive equipment and a deep plane of anesthesia. Samples obtained from a transoral wash may be cultured for bacteria and viruses, and may be evaluated for bacteria, neoplastic cells, fungal infection, or parasitic organisms or ova. The samples obtained from a transoral wash may be reflective of large airways, and, unlike those obtained from a BAL, may not be reflective of what is deep within the alveoli of the lung(s).

Supplies Needed

Sterile endotracheal tube
Sterile saline
Sterile red rubber catheter or polypropylene rigid urinary catheter
12-ml syringes (sterile)
Port-a–Cul™ culture swabs
Lavender- and red-topped vials

Indications

Obtain bacterial or viral cultures from airway
Obtain cells for cytologic evaluation of airway

Contraindications

Condition in which light-plane general anesthesia is determined to be too dangerous in a very fragile patient

Limitations

Samples obtained may be more reflective of large airways, and not reflective of what is deeper in the lung(s)

 Video available online

Go to www.wiley.com/go/hackett to view a video of this procedure.

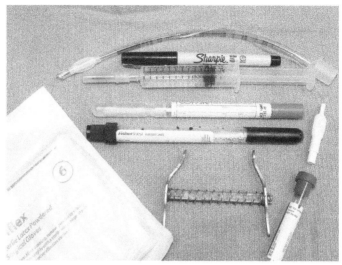

Fig. 4.36. Supplies required for sample collection via transoral wash.

Helpful hint: Have all supplies necessary prepared and in place before placing the patient under anesthesia.

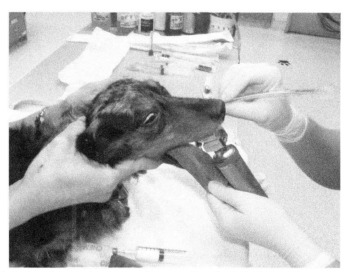

Fig. 4.37. After induction of anesthesia, pass a sterile, new endotracheal tube in as sterile a manner as possible. Have flow-by oxygen available, and be prepared to breathe for the patient in between airway washes.

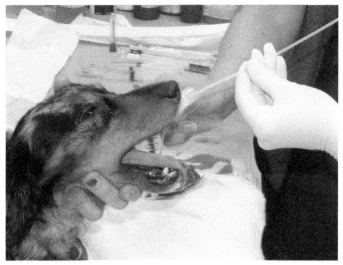

Fig. 4.38. Pass a rigid polypropylene or red rubber catheter into the patient's airway, through the endotracheal tube.

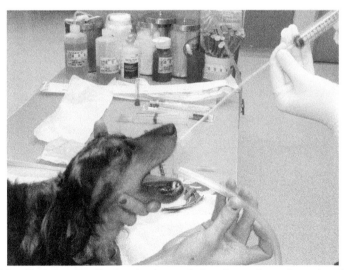

Fig. 4.39. Instill 5 to 10 ml of sterile saline into the airways via the polypropylene catheter, then vigorously coupage or tap the patient's lateral thorax.

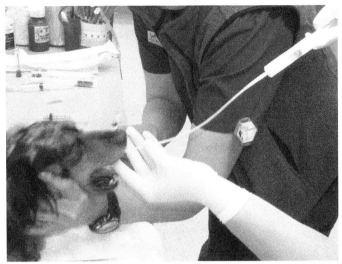

Fig. 4.40. Withdraw the fluid from the polypropylene catheter. Note: Not all fluid that was instilled will be withdrawn from the airways.

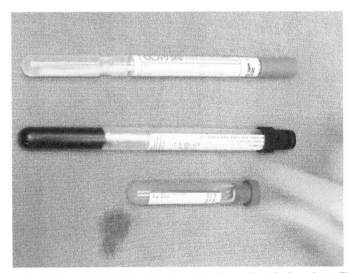

Fig. 4.41. Save samples of airway fluid for bacterial and/or viral culture and cytologic analyses. This entire process can be repeated up to a total of three times.

TRANSTHORACIC ASPIRATE

Introduction

Transthoracic aspirate is an easy, inexpensive technique for obtaining diagnostic samples from discrete lesions within the pulmonary parenchyma. It is simply a fine needle aspirate of parenchymal tissue. Transthoracic aspirate may be considered in any patient with nodular, interstitial, or discrete mass lesions within the lung tissue.

The site of the aspirate is determined by close examination of lateral and dorso-ventral (or ventro-dorsal) radiographs of the chest. Having perpendicular radiographic views allows lesion location and depth to be assessed.

The procedure carries a risk of iatrogenic pneumothorax. Transthoracic aspiration should be quick and the patient monitored closely for signs of respiratory distress. On some occasions a patient may have to be managed for pneumothorax after the procedure is performed. This complication should be discussed with the owner before the procedure and the risks/benefits considered for each patient.

Disposable spinal needles with an internal stylet are preferred for this procedure to avoid introducing tissue from the skin and chest wall to the sample.

Supplies Needed

20- to 22-gauge, 1–1/2 to 2–1/2 spinal needle long enough to reach the lesion or 20- to
    22-gauge, 1–1/2-inch needles
6- to 12-cc syringe
Clippers and blades
Nonsterile gloves
Aseptic scrub
Microscope slides
Port-a-Cul™ for bacterial culture

Indications

Diagnosis of pulmonary parenchymal disorders not amenable to trans-airway wash or bronchoscopy. Common examples include nodular interstitial diseases (neoplasia, fungal infections) and mass lesions.

Cautions and Contraindications

Caution must be exercised because the risk of iatrogenic pneumothorax increases with every breath the patient takes while the needle is in the lung parenchyma.

 Video available online

Go to www.wiley.com/go/hackett to view a video of this procedure.

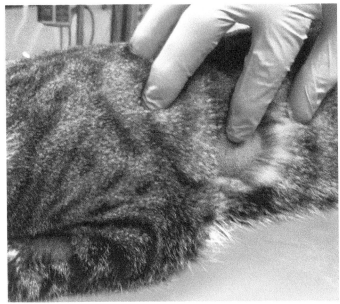

Fig. 4.42. After reviewing thoracic radiographs, the location and depth of the area of interest is identified on the patient. The hair is clipped over the site and the skin prepped for aseptic aspiration.

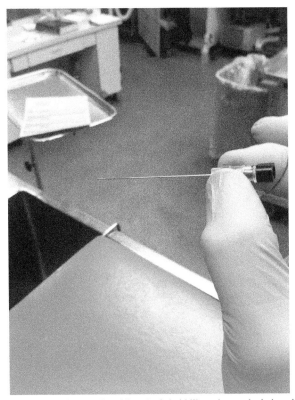

Fig. 4.43. A 22-gauge, 2–1/2-inch spinal needle with stylet is held like a dart so the hub and depth can be clearly seen during insertion.

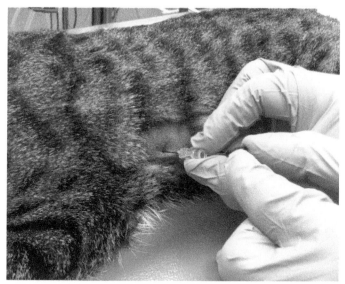

Fig. 4.44. The needle and stylet are inserted quickly. To avoid cytologic contamination with skin and chest wall tissue, the stylet is only removed once the needle has reached the pre-determined depth.

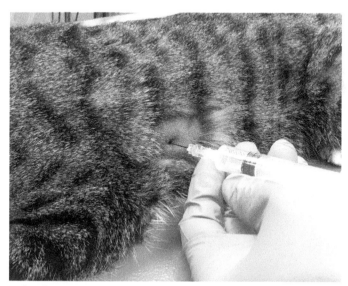

Fig. 4.45. A 6-cc syringe is attached to the spinal needle and quickly aspirated two to three times. The syringe is allowed to return to a neutral position so as not to maintain negative pressure while the needle is withdrawn. This will prevent sample contamination.

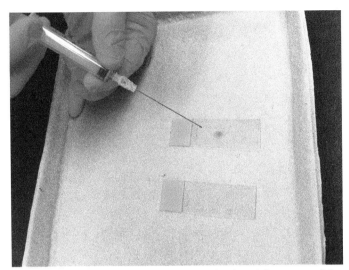

Fig. 4.46. The syringe is briefly removed from the needle, filled with air, and the contents of the needle expelled onto a clean glass slide. A pull prep is made and the slide fixed and stained for cytologic evaluation.

REFERENCES

Hedlund CS. Surgery of the Upper Respiratory System. In: Fossum TW (Ed): *Small Animal Surgery*. St. Louis: Mosby. pp. 613–614, 1997.

Macintire DK, Drobatz KJ, Haskins SC, Saxon WD. Respiratory Emergencies. In: *Manual of Small Animal Emergency and Critical Care Medicine*. Philadelphia: Lippincott, Williams and Wilkins. pp. 115–119, 2005.

Marks SL. Nasal oxygen insufflation. *J Amer Anim Hosp Assoc* 35:366, 1999.

Murtaugh RJ. Acute respiratory distress. *Vet Clin North Amer Sm Anim* 24(6):1041–1055, 1994.

Raffee MR. Respiratory Care. In: Wingfield WE, Raffee M (Eds): *The Veterinary ICU Book*. Jackson, WY: Teton NewMedia. pp. 147–165, 2002.

CHAPTER 5

Urinary Catheter Placement, Urohydropulsion, and Temporary Antepubic Cystostomy Catheter Placement

URINARY CATHETER PLACEMENT IN MALE AND FEMALE DOGS

Introduction

Placement of a urinary catheter often serves a dual purpose in critically ill small animal patients. In non-ambulatory animals, a urinary catheter attached to a closed collection system is invaluable in maintaining cleanliness and preventing urine scald and decubital ulceration. Urine collection and quantitation is often necessary when assessing perfusion parameters and renal function. Finally, urethral catheterization and maintenance of an indwelling urinary catheter is necessary in the treatment of urethral obstruction in cases of feline lower urinary tract disease and urethral calculi. This chapter describes the placement of various types of urinary catheters in male and female dogs and cats.

Supplies Needed

Electric clippers and blades
Sterile gloves
Antimicrobial scrub and solution
1-inch white tape
20- to 30-ml syringe
Sterile 0.9% saline solution
Sterile needle holder
Sterile huck towels
Urine collection bag
Sterile IV infusion line
Sterile lubricating jelly

Veterinary Emergency and Critical Care Procedures, Second Edition. Timothy B. Hackett and Elisa M. Mazzaferro.
© 2012 John Wiley & Sons, Inc. Published 2012 by John Wiley & Sons, Inc.

Christmas tree adapter
Vaginal speculum
Sterile otoscope head
Light source
3–0 nonabsorbable suture
Foley catheter
Red rubber catheter
Infant feeding tube

Indications

Maintenance of patient cleanliness in nonambulatory patients
Urine collection for urinalysis
Urine quantitation
Treatment of urethral obstruction
Urethral trauma
Urethral prolapse

Contraindications

Not indicated in patients that are ambulatory and do not have urinary obstruction, or do not require urine quantitation.

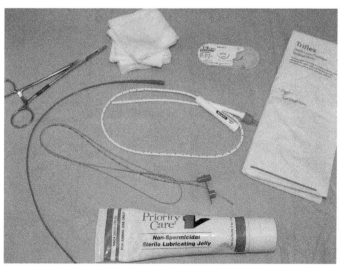

Fig. 5.1. Supplies needed for placement of a urinary catheter differ for males and females. Required supplies include electric clippers and blades, antimicrobial scrub and solution, sterile 0.9% saline, 20- to 30-ml sterile syringes, 1-inch white tape, 3- to 6-ml syringes, sterile needle holder, sterile field/huck towels, urinary catheter, sterile lubricating jelly, Christmas tree adapter, light source, and 3–0 nonabsorbable suture. For female urinary catheter placement, a vaginal speculum or otoscope with a sterile head and light source may come in handy.

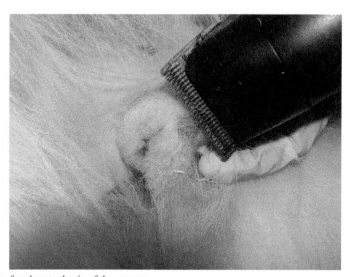

Fig. 5.2. Clip the fur close to the tip of the prepuce.

Helpful hint: Use caution to not cause skin irritation.

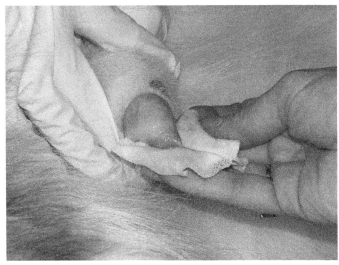

Fig. 5.3. Scrub the tip of the prepuce with antimicrobial scrub and solution. Extrude the penis and scrub the tip of the penis in a similar manner.

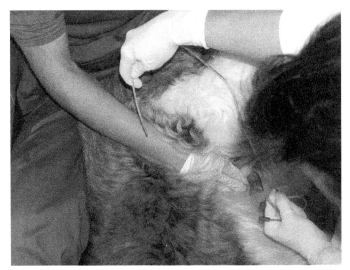

Fig. 5.4. Wearing sterile gloves, measure the catheter from the tip of the penis to the urinary bladder. This is to ensure that you don't insert the catheter too far, causing it to coil on itself and making removal difficult or impossible.

Helpful hint: Use care to not contaminate the catheter by touching it to the patient's fur.

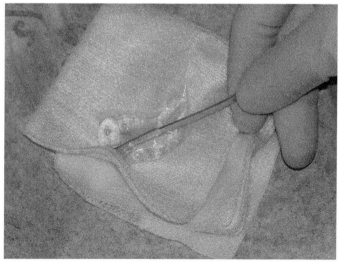

Fig. 5.5. Wearing sterile gloves, lubricate the tip of the urinary catheter and gently insert it into the distal urethra.

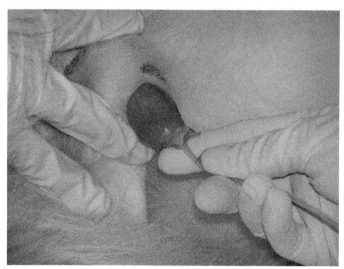

Fig. 5.6. Continue to insert the catheter to the appropriate length.

Helpful hint: Once the catheter is in the urinary bladder, urine should flow freely from the catheter. Use caution if a urinary bladder rupture is suspected, because urine may not flow readily due to leakage into the abdominal cavity.

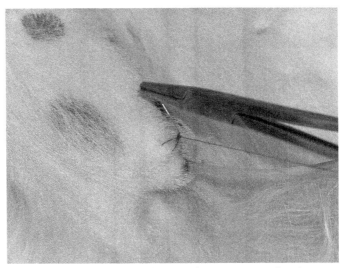

Fig. 5.7. Attach the catheter to a closed system for urine collection. You can now allow the prepuce to fall back into its normal position. Place two stay sutures in the tip of the prepuce. This step can be avoided if you use a Foley catheter.

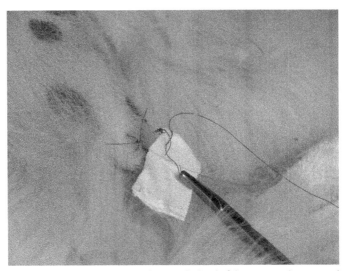

Fig. 5.8. Place a length of white tape around the catheter at the level of the prepuce, then suture the white tape to the stay sutures to secure the catheter in place.

Helpful hint: Make sure that the catheter is completely dry and the tape is securely fastened on the catheter, or else the catheter will slip out.

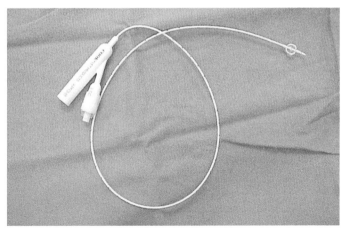

Fig. 5.9. Alternate technique if a Foley catheter is used: After routinely aseptically preparing the prepuce and penis as directed above, lubricate the tip of a Foley catheter with sterile lubricant, and insert it into the penis and urinary bladder as previously described. Inflate the bladder of the Foley catheter with the appropriate amount of sterile saline solution. Gently pull the urinary catheter out until you feel slight resistance as the balloon at the end of the catheter goes snugly into place.

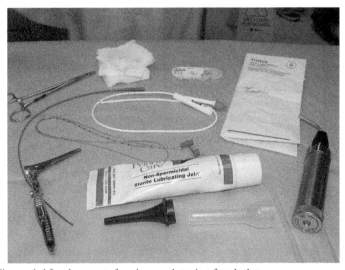

Fig. 5.10. Supplies needed for placement of a urinary catheter in a female dog.

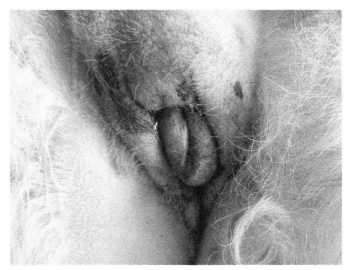

Fig. 5.11. Gently clip the fur from the vulva.

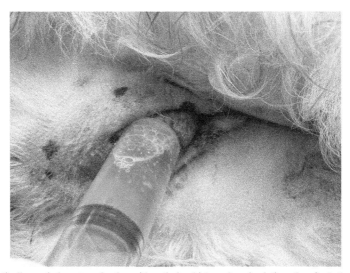

Fig. 5.12. Aseptically scrub the external vulva with antimicrobial scrub and solution, then flush the vulva with dilute antimicrobial solution mixed with 0.9% saline or sterile water.

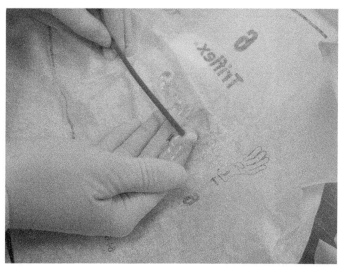

Fig. 5.13. Wearing sterile gloves, lubricate the tip of the sterile urinary catheter with sterile lubricant or lidocaine jelly.

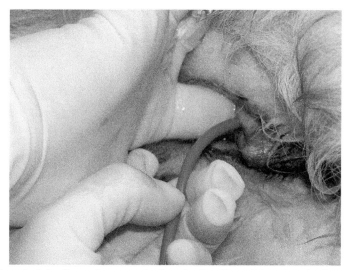

Fig. 5.14. Lubricate the index finger of your non-dominant hand, and insert it into the patient's vagina. Palpate for the urethral papilla on the ventral floor of the vagina.

Helpful hint: Curve the tip of your index finger ventrally, so that once you insert the catheter into the vagina, the catheter will "dip" toward the ventral vaginal floor and slide into the urethra.

(a)

(b)

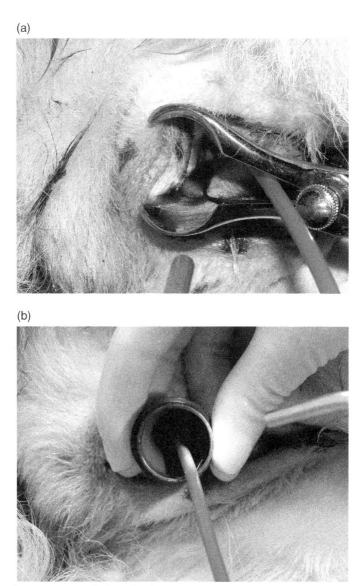

Figs. 5.15a–b. If you are unsuccessful in performing the "blind" catheterization technique, you can lubricate and insert a sterile vaginal speculum, sterile otoscope head, or sterile 6-ml syringe case into the vagina and visualize the urethral papilla to facilitate catheter insertion.

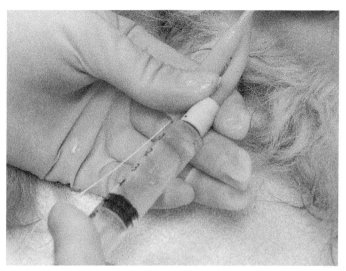

Fig. 5.16. If a Foley catheter is used, insert sterile saline to fill the balloon at the catheter tip.

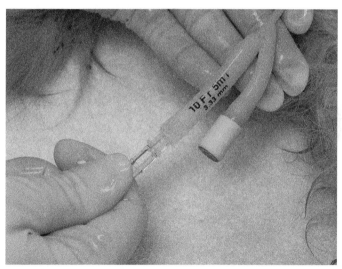

Fig. 5.17. Urine will flow from the catheter once it has been successfully introduced into the urinary bladder. In rare cases, no urine will flow if the bladder is completely empty or if the bladder has ruptured.

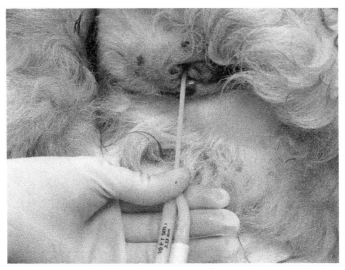

Fig. 5.18. Attach the catheter to a closed urine collection system after you observe urine flowing.

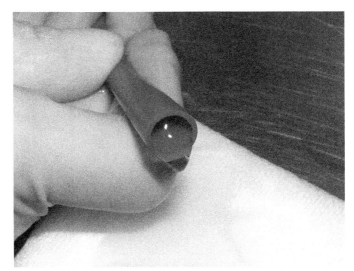

Fig. 5.19. Gently pull on the urinary catheter until you feel slight resistance as the balloon becomes seated snugly in the urinary bladder.

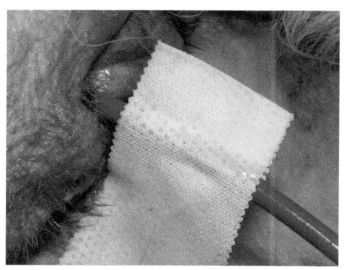

Fig. 5.20. If a Foley catheter was not used, place two stay sutures on either side of the vulva, then attach a length of 1-inch white adhesive tape to the catheter.

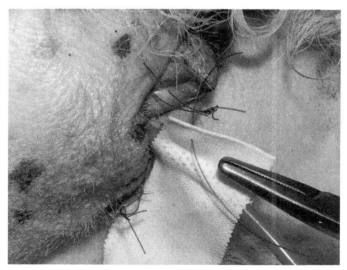

Fig. 5.21. Suture the white tape to the stay sutures, and then gently secure the catheter to the base of the tail with 1-inch white adhesive tape.

Helpful hint: Make sure that the catheter is completely dry and that the tape is secured firmly to the catheter or the catheter can slip.

URETHRAL CATHETERIZATION IN MALE AND FEMALE CATS

Supplies Needed

Sterile gloves
Antimicrobial scrub
3-, 6-, 12-, 20-ml sterile syringes
Sterile lubricating jelly
Sterile 0.9% saline solution
Closed-end Tomcat catheter
Argyle 3 French and 5 French infant feeding tube or red rubber catheters
1-inch white adhesive tape
3–0 nonabsorbable suture
Urine collection bag
Sterile catheter adapter
Sterile IV infusion tubing

 | Video available online

Go to www.wiley.com/go/hackett to view a video of this procedure.

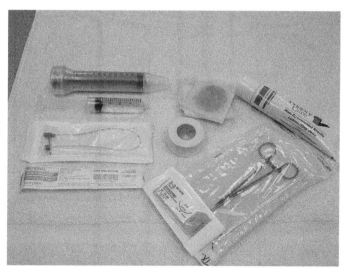

Fig. 5.22. Supplies needed for feline urethral catheterization.

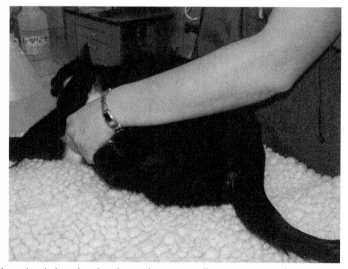

Fig. 5.23. Lay the patient in lateral or dorsal recumbency, according to operator preference.

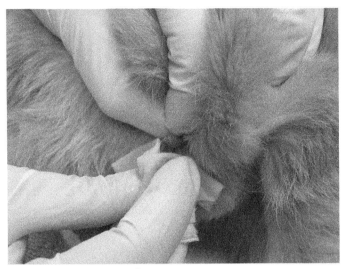

Fig. 5.24. Aseptically scrub the prepuce and penis.

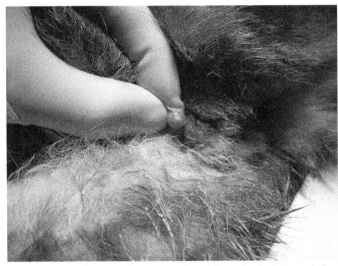

Fig. 5.25. Wearing sterile gloves, reflect the tail dorsally and cranially, and extrude the penis from the prepuce, grasping the prepuce tightly at the base of the penis between your thumb and index finger. This prevents the prepuce from slipping back over the penis. Alternatively, the penis can be grasped with a 1 × 2 rat tooth forceps. After the penis is extruded, palpate the tip and examine the distal urethra for a calculus or crystal debris that may be the source of obstruction.

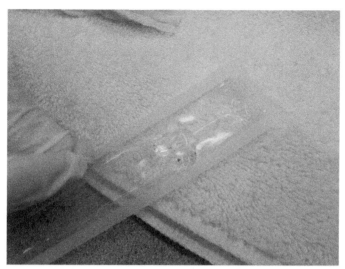

Fig. 5.26. Lubricate the tip of the Tomcat catheter with sterile lubricating jelly.

Helpful hint: Keep a couple of Tomcat catheters in the freezer. Freezing will cause them to become more rigid, and will help facilitate urethral catheterization.

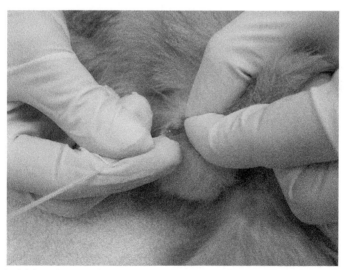

Fig. 5.27. Insert the lubricated catheter into the urethra and advance as far as possible. Note: If the catheter will not advance, follow the instructions the hydropulsion section below.

Helpful hint: You may feel a "gritty" sensation if urethral calculi are present.

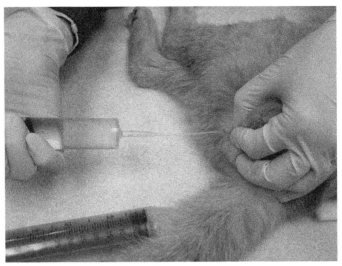

Fig. 5.28. Once the urinary catheter is in place, flush the urinary bladder until the urine comes back clear.

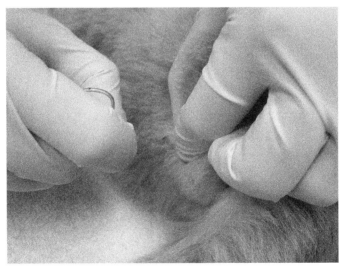

Fig. 5.29. Remove the rigid Tomcat catheter and replace with a flexible Argyle infant feeding tube or 3 French or 5 French red rubber catheter.

Helpful hint: Make sure to measure the catheter first to prevent putting too much of the catheter into the urinary bladder. Use care to not contaminate the catheter by touching it to the patient's fur.

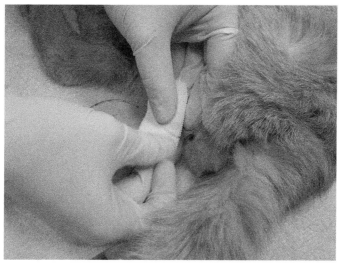

Fig. 5.30. Dry off the catheter, and place a length of 1-inch white adhesive tape around the catheter at the level of the prepuce.

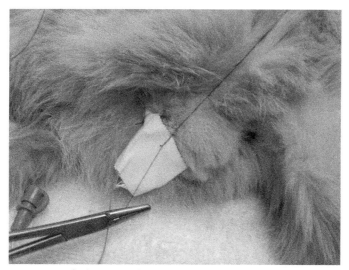

Fig. 5.31. Place two stay sutures in the prepuce. Suture the adhesive tape to the stay sutures.

Helpful hint: Make sure to not kink the catheter, because this will cause obstruction.

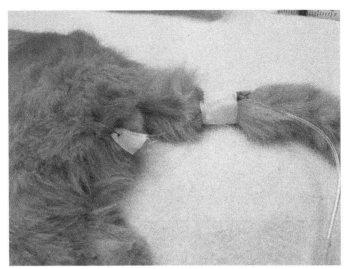

Fig. 5.32. Attach the catheter to a closed collection system. Attach the catheter to the tail with a length of white adhesive tape.

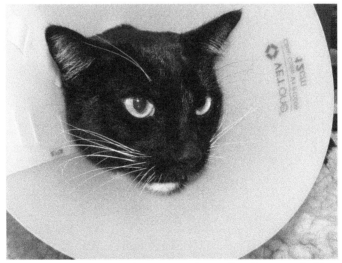

Fig. 5.33. Place an Elizabethan collar on the patient to prevent iatrogenic patient removal of the catheter.

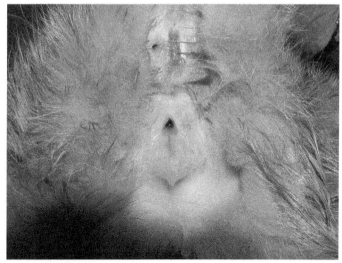

Fig. 5.34. Urinary catheter placement in the female cat. Place the patient in lateral or sternal recumbency, according to operator preference. The equipment required is the same as for a male cat urinary catheter.

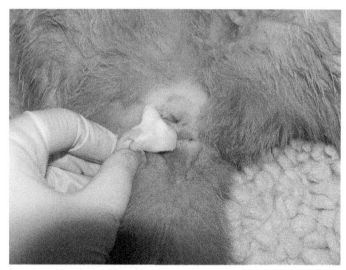

Fig. 5.35. Scrub the vulva with antimicrobial scrub.

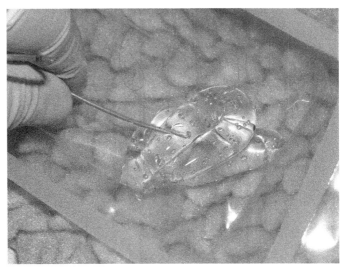

Fig. 5.36. Wearing sterile gloves, lubricate the tip of an Argyle infant feeding catheter or red rubber catheter that has been placed in the freezer to make it more rigid.

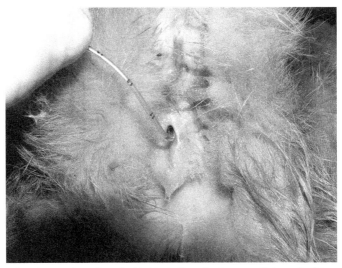

Fig. 5.37. Measure the urinary catheter from the bladder to the vulva to ensure that you don't insert the catheter too far. Insert the tip of the catheter into the ventral vulva, and push cranially as you pull the edges of the vulva caudally. The catheter tip should slip into the urethral papilla and then into the urinary bladder. Placement is confirmed by aspirating urine from the catheter.

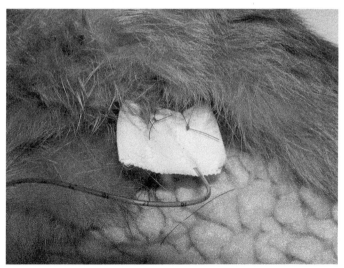

Fig. 5.38. Attach a length of 1-inch white adhesive tape to the catheter just adjacent to the vulva. Place two stay sutures on either side of the vulva using non-absorbable suture. Suture the adhesive tape to the stay sutures.

Helpful hint: Use caution to not kink the catheter, because this could cause mechanical obstruction.

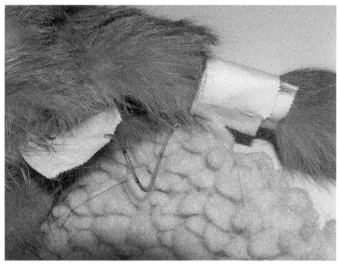

Fig. 5.39. Attach the end of the catheter to a closed collection system for urine quantitation, and then tape the tubing to the tail.

UROHYDROPULSION

Introduction

Urohydropulsion is a procedure that is sometimes required to pass a urethral catheter in a male dog that has urethral calculi causing obstruction. In most cases, the patient must be heavily sedated or placed under general anesthesia to minimize discomfort and optimize successful catheter placement. The goal of urohydropulsion is to push a urethral calculus back into the urinary bladder until definitive removal via cystotomy can be performed. The supplies required for urohydropulsion are the same as for placement of a urinary catheter.

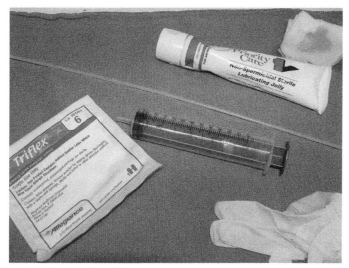

Fig. 5.40. Supplies needed for urohydropulsion.

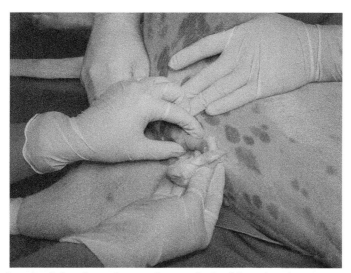

Fig. 5.41. Place the patient in lateral recumbency and prepare the tip of the penis and prepuce as previously described.

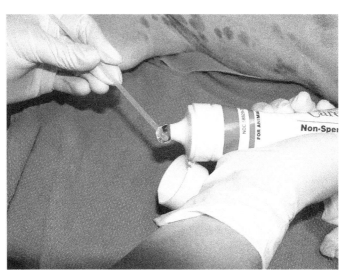

Fig. 5.42. Lubricate the catheter tip with sterile lubricant.

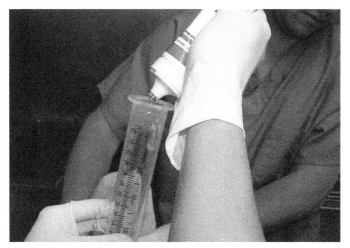

Fig. 5.43. Place a small amount of sterile lubricant and sterile saline into a 20-ml syringe.

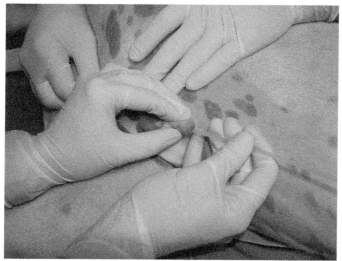

Fig. 5.44. Insert sterile lubricant jelly and sterile saline solution mixture into the tip of the penis with a rigid catheter.

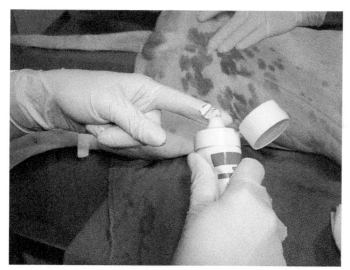

Fig. 5.45. Have an assistant lubricate her gloved index finger.

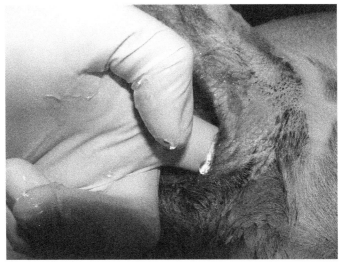

Fig. 5.46. Have the assistant insert her gloved index finger into the patient's rectum and push ventrally on the floor of the rectum to occlude the urethra as it passes over the floor of the pelvis.

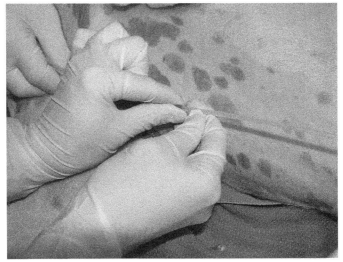

Fig. 5.47. Pinch the distal penis closely around the catheter between your thumb and index finger.

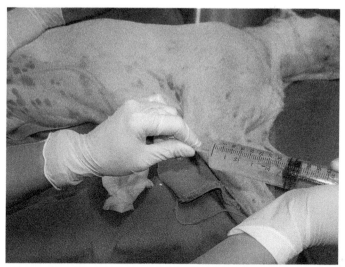

Fig. 5.48. Using a 20-ml syringe, inject and pulse the mixture of sterile saline and sterile lubricant into the catheter as the assistant pushes up and down on the pelvic urethra. This technique will alternately increase and decrease the pressure in the urethra to dislodge the urethral calculus and retropulse it back into the urinary bladder. Pass the urinary catheter and secure it in place until removal of the calculus can be performed.

TEMPORARY ANTEPUBLIC CYSTOSTOMY CATHETER PLACEMENT

Introduction and Indications

When urethral catheterization is impossible and the patient is too unstable to perform a cystotomy or perineal urethrostomy due to electrolyte and acid-base derangements, the placement of a temporary antepubic cystostomy catheter using local anesthesia can be life-saving to keep the urinary bladder drained until electrolyte and acid-base disturbances are normalized.

Supplies Needed

Foley balloon-tipped catheter
2% lidocaine
Electric clippers and blades
Antimicrobial scrub
Sterile huck towels
Towel clamps
Number 10 and 11 scalpel blades
Kelly hemostats
Mettzenbaum scissors
Absorbable suture
Nonabsorbable suture

Contraindications

Urethral catheterization is possible
Pyometra
Transitional cell carcinoma of the urinary bladder

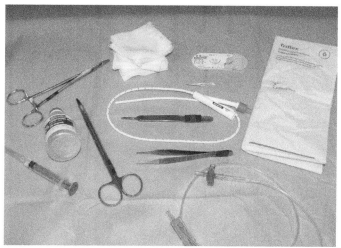

Fig. 5.49. Supplies needed for temporary antepubic cystostomy catheter.

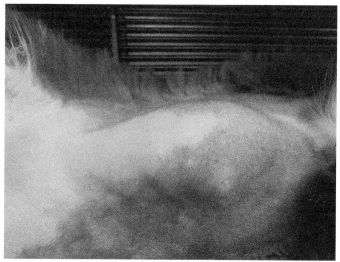

Fig. 5.50. Place the patient in dorsal recumbency and clip the ventral midline from the umbilicus to the pubis and laterally to the folds of the flank.

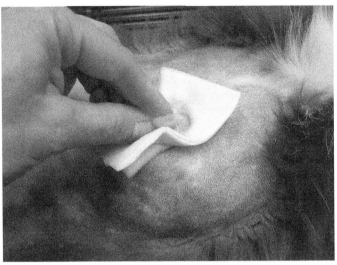

Fig. 5.51. Aseptically scrub the clipped area, then drape with sterile towels secured with towel clamps.

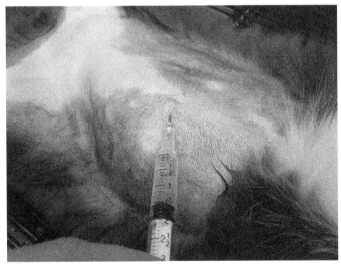

Fig. 5.52. Wearing sterile gloves, tent the skin over the urinary bladder in between your thumb and index finger, and inject 2% lidocaine in to the level of the peritoneum, injecting the local anesthetic as you withdraw the needle.

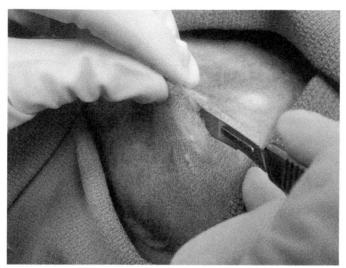

Fig. 5.53. Make a small stab incision into the anesthetized area with a number 10 scalpel blade.

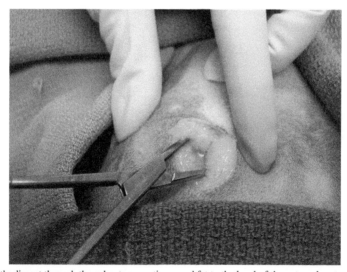

Fig. 5.54. Bluntly dissect through the subcutaneous tissue and fat to the level of the external rectus abdominus muscles. Visualize the linea alba in midline.

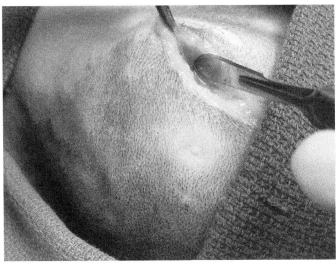

Fig. 5.55. Pick up the linea alba over the urinary bladder with a thumb forceps and make a small stab incision.

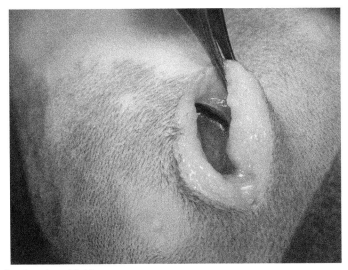

Fig. 5.56. Visualize the urinary bladder.

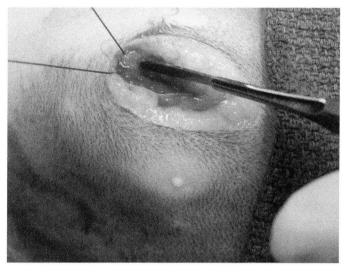

Fig. 5.57. Place a purse-string suture through the urinary bladder; leave the ends long to allow you to retract the urinary bladder to the level of the skin as you insert the urinary catheter. Make a small stab incision into the urinary bladder with a number 11 scalpel blade.

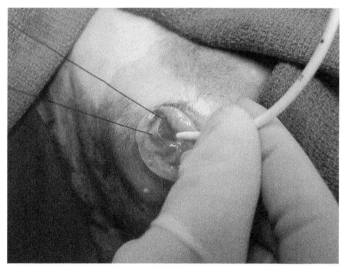

Fig. 5.58. Insert the Foley catheter through the incision in the urinary bladder, and then inflate the balloon with the appropriate amount of sterile saline. Pull the urinary bladder snugly against the body wall while you suture the linea, subcutaneous tissues, and skin.

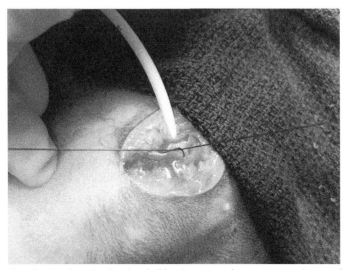

Fig. 5.59. Secure the urinary catheter in place by cinching the purse-string suture securely around the tube and tying in place. Snip the ends of the suture short.

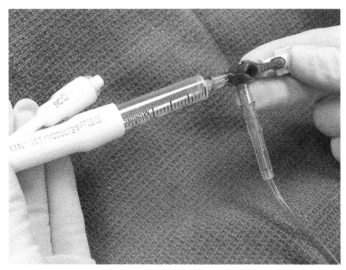

Fig. 5.60. Connect the catheter to a closed urine collection system using a sterile catheter adapter.

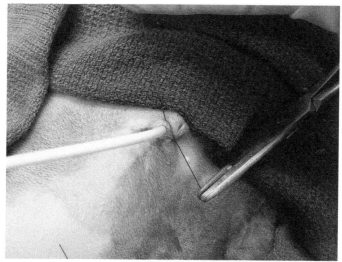

Fig. 5.61. Close the subcutaneous tissues with absorbable suture, then close the skin with a purse-string suture of non-absorbable suture. Leave the ends of the suture long, and secure them in a finger-trap suture around the urinary catheter. Place triple antibiotic ointment over the place of catheter insertion, and cover with 4-×4-inch sterile gauze squares. Bandage the catheter in place to the ventral abdomen with cotton roll gauze, Kling, and Vetrap™ or ElastiKon®. Make sure to label the location of the catheter to prevent you from accidentally cutting it later during a routine bandage change.

REFERENCES

Battaglia AM. Urogenital emergencies. In: *Small Animal Emergency and Critical Care: A Manual for the Veterinary Technician*. Philadelphia: W.B. Saunders. 2001.

Crow SE, Walshaw, SO. Urethral catheterization. In: *Manual of Clinical Procedures in the Dog and Cat*. Philadelphia: J.B. Lippincott Company. pp. 110–127, 1987.

Hayashi K, Hardie RJ. Use of cystostomy tubes in small animals. *Compend Contin Educ Pract Vet* 25(12):928, 934, 2003.

Salinardi BJ, Marks SL, Davidson JR, Senior DF. The use of a low-profile cystostomy tube to relieve urethral obstruction in a dog. *J Amer Anim Hosp Assoc* 39(4):403–405, 2003.

Smarick S. Urinary Catheterization. In: Silverstein DC, Hopper K (Eds): *Small Animal Critical Care Medicine*. St. Louis: Saunders-Elsevier. pp. 603–606, 2009.

CHAPTER 6

Abdominocentesis and Diagnostic Peritoneal Lavage

ABDOMINOCENTESIS

Introduction

Abdominal paracentesis (abdominocentesis) is a useful and inexpensive technique to identify abdominal effusion, particularly in patients with clinical signs of acute abdominal pain or unexplained fever. Evaluation of any fluid obtained often aids in the diagnosis and helps guide treatment. Abdominal effusion can be classified according to its cellularity and protein content as transudates, modified transudates, and exudates. Causes of modified transudates and exudates include neoplasia, septic and non-septic inflammation, and hemorrhage. Additionally, biochemical evaluation of the fluid for blood urea nitrogen, creatinine, potassium, amylase, lipase, bilirubin, and glucose can aid in the diagnosis of various conditions, including uroabdomen, pancreatitis, bile peritonitis, and septic peritonitis.

Supplies Needed

20- to 22-gauge, 1- to 1–1/2-inch needles
Latex gloves
Electric clipper and blades
3- to 6-ml syringes
Antimicrobial scrub
Sterile EDTA and red-topped tubes
Port-A-Cul™ sterile culturettes for bacterial isolation

Veterinary Emergency and Critical Care Procedures, Second Edition. Timothy B. Hackett and Elisa M. Mazzaferro.
© 2012 John Wiley & Sons, Inc. Published 2012 by John Wiley & Sons, Inc.

Indications

Diagnosis and treatment of hemoabdomen, uroabdomen, bile or septic peritonitis, and/or
neoplastic effusions

Contraindications

Penetrating abdominal wounds (exploratory laparotomy required)

Limitations

Is insensitive in the diagnosis of retroperitoneal effusions (hemorrhage, urinary tract leakage,
neoplasia, abscess) Limitations of this technique are a false negative abdominocentesis
if small (<7 ml/kg) amounts of abdominal effusion are present.

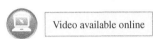 Video available online

Go to www.wiley.com/go/hackett to view a video of this procedure.

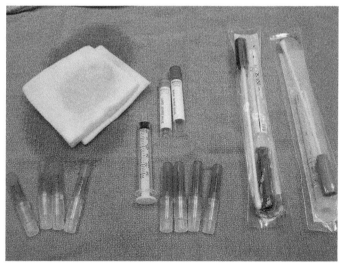

Fig. 6.1. Equipment needed for abdominocentesis.

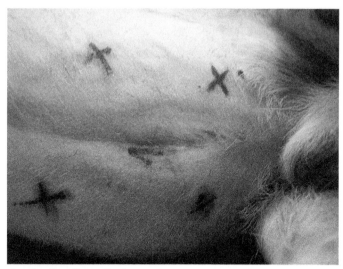

Fig. 6.2. Four quadrant locations for needle placement.

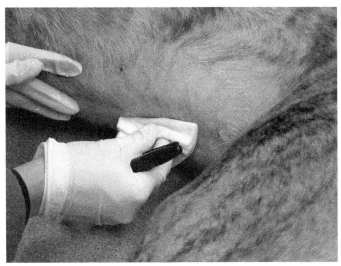

Fig. 6.3. Clip and aseptically scrub a 10-cm square area of the ventral abdomen with the umbilicus in the center of the clipped area.

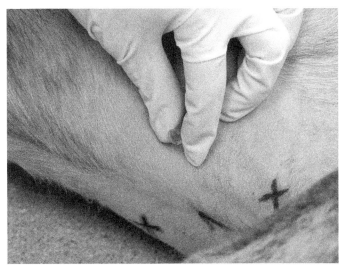

Fig. 6.4. Insert the needle cranial and to the right of the umbilicus, twisting gently as the needle is inserted into the peritoneal cavity to push any hollow organ away from the tip of the needle. If fluid does not flow freely, repeat insertion of the needle as described in the following locations: to the left and cranial, to the right and caudal, and to the left and caudal to the umbilicus.

Helpful hint: In some cases, fluid will not flow freely until a second needle is inserted into the peritoneal cavity.

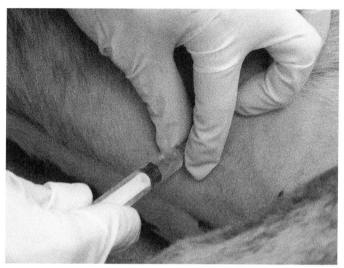

Fig. 6.5. Gently aspirate fluid if fluid does not flow freely.

Helpful hint: Abdominocentesis may be falsely NEGATIVE with this technique if less than 5 to 7 ml/kg of fluid are present within the peritoneal cavity.

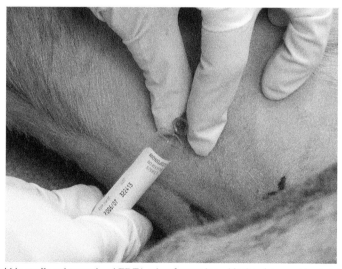

Fig. 6.6. Save fluid in sterile red-topped and EDTA tubes for cytology, biochemistry, and bacterial analyses.

DIAGNOSTIC PERITONEAL LAVAGE

Introduction and Indications

Diagnostic peritoneal lavage (DPL) can be performed in patients with acute abdominal pain and unexplained fever when four-quadrant abdominocentesis is negative. DPL is more sensitive when small amounts of abdominal effusion are present, and when there is rupture of a hollow viscus, particularly after blunt or penetrating trauma. DPL also can be used to identify and evaluate the character of abdominal effusion post-operatively.

Supplies Needed

20- to 22-gauge, 1- to 1-1/2 inch needles OR
16- to 20-gauge, 1-1/2-inch over-the-needle catheter
Sterile glass red- and purple-topped tubes for sample collection
3- to 6-ml syringes
Electric clippers and fresh blades
Antimicrobial scrub
Warm (37°C) isotonic crystalloid fluid (Normosol®-R, Lactated Ringer's, 0.9% saline)
Intravenous fluid administration set
Rapid infusion IV pressure bag
Sterile gloves, field towels (4)
Backhaus towel clamps
Optional supplies: Over-the-wire diagnostic peritoneal lavage kit

Indications

Identification and characterization of small amounts of abdominal effusion when abdominal paracentesis is negative

Contraindications

Penetrating injury to the abdominal cavity that requires exploratory laparotomy

Limitations

Is insensitive in the diagnosis of retroperitoneal effusions (hemorrhage, urinary tract leakage, neoplasia, abscess). A limitation of this technique is that any fluid collected must be interpreted carefully, because dilution of total cell count and chemical analysis always occurs.

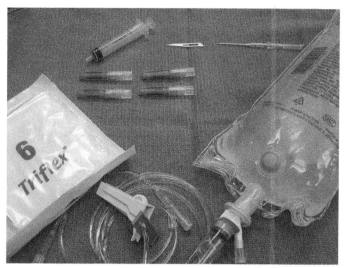

Fig. 6.7. Equipment needed for diagnostic peritoneal lavage.

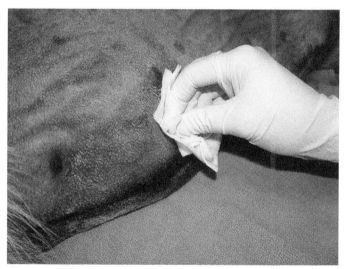

Fig. 6.8. Place the patient in lateral recumbency and clip and aseptically scrub a 10-cm area of the ventral abdomen, with the umbilicus in the center. Drape the clipped area with sterile field towels secured with towel clamps.

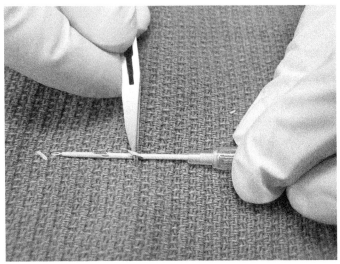

Fig. 6.9. Wearing sterile gloves, use a number 10 scalpel blade to fenestrate side-ports in an over-the-needle catheter.

Helpful hint: Use care to avoid making a hole greater than 50% the circumference of the catheter. A large hole will weaken the catheter and increase the risk of breaking off into the peritoneal cavity.

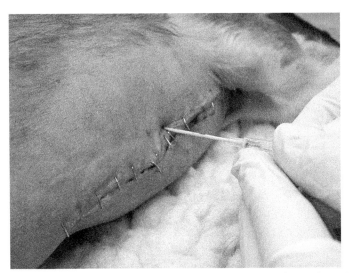

Fig. 6.10. Wearing sterile gloves, insert the over-the-needle catheter into the abdominal cavity caudal and to the right of the umbilicus, at the level of the nipples. Advance the catheter slowly and with a gentle twisting motion to avoid iatrogenic puncture of any abdominal organs.

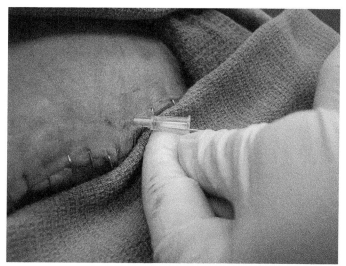

Fig. 6.11. Withdraw the stylette from the catheter, and examine the catheter hub for the presence of any fluid. If fluid is present, withdraw the fluid using a sterile 3-ml syringe.

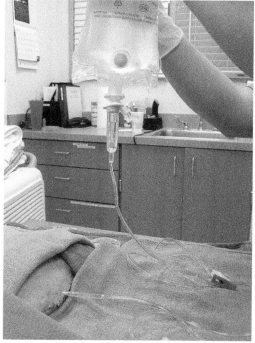

Fig. 6.12. If no fluid is present, instill 10 to 20 ml/kg of warmed Lactated Ringer's or 0.9% saline solution into the abdominal cavity over a period of three to five minutes. Watch the patient carefully for the presence of discomfort or respiratory difficulty; if that occurs, abandon the fluid infusion.

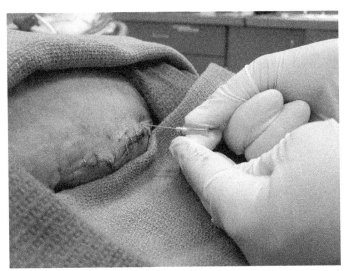

Fig. 6.13. Remove the catheter, and gently roll the patient from side to side or allow an ambulatory patient to walk while you massage the abdomen to redistribute the fluid that you have just infused into the abdominal cavity. Lay the patient in lateral recumbency and aseptically prepare the abdomen to perform a four-quadrant abdominocentesis. Ideally, remove at least 0.5 to 1 ml of the lavage fluid to analyze for cytology and culture.

Helpful hint: In most cases, the majority of the fluid you have infused will not be recovered. Only small amounts of the infused fluid will be recovered for analyses. Any biochemical analyses performed will be diluted if a diagnostic peritoneal lavage has been performed.

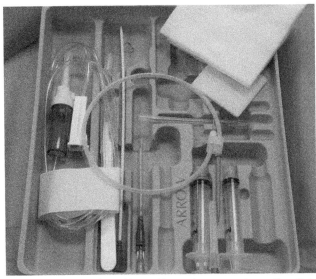

Fig. 6.14. The over-the-wire diagnostic peritoneal lavage kit contains an over-the-needle catheter and hypodermic needle through which to insert the J-wire into the abdominal cavity, J-wire, and peritoneal lavage catheter. Depending on the manufacturer, some kits also contain gauze, a scalpel blade, syringes, and an infusion set.

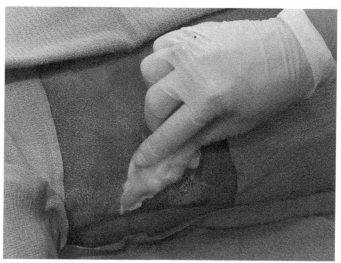

Fig. 6.15. Clip and aseptically scrub the patient's ventral abdomen, then drape the area with sterile field towels or surgical drape material.

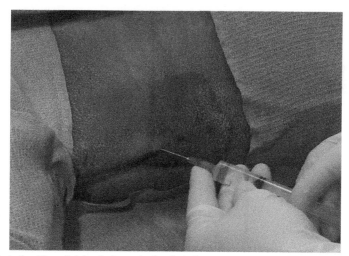

Fig. 6.16. Infiltrate the skin and abdominal muscles just lateral to the umbilicus with 1 mg/kg 2% lidocaine (0.5 mg/kg in cats).

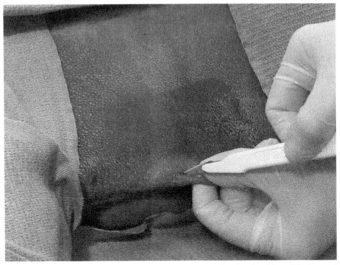

Fig. 6.17. Tent the skin over the anesthetized area, and make a small nick in the skin with the scalpel blade.

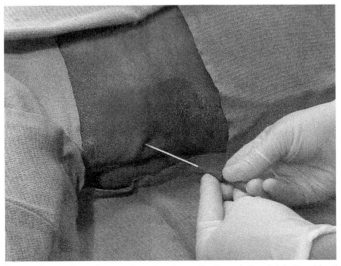

Fig. 6.18. Insert the over-the-needle catheter or hypodermic needle through the nick in the skin, through the abdominal muscles, and into the peritoneal cavity. Twist as the needle penetrates into the peritoneal cavity to push any hollow viscera away from the needle.

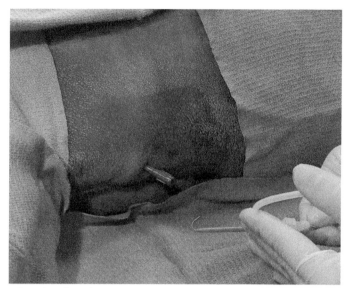

Fig. 6.19. Remove the stylette from the catheter. Retract the J-wire into its sheath. Insert the J-wire adapter into the catheter or hypodermic hub.

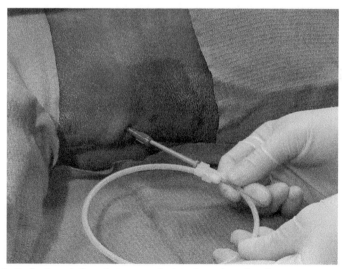

Fig. 6.20. Push the J-wire through the catheter or needle, into the peritoneal cavity.

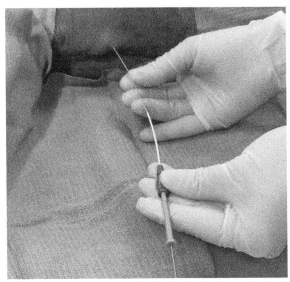

Fig. 6.21. Remove the catheter or hypodermic needle off of the J-wire, leaving the J-wire in place within the peritoneal cavity.

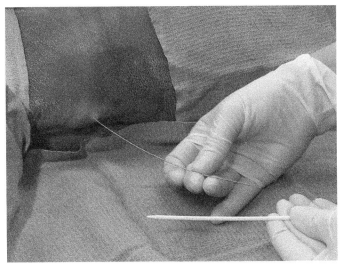

Fig. 6.22. Next, pass the diagnostic peritoneal lavage catheter over the J-wire, into the peritoneal cavity. Note the multiple holes in the catheter to facilitate lavage.

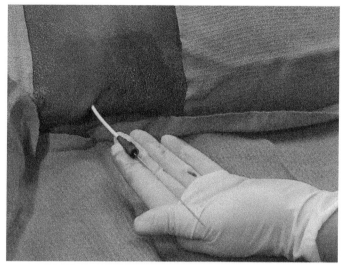

Fig. 6.23. The catheter can be inserted into the peritoneal cavity to its hub.

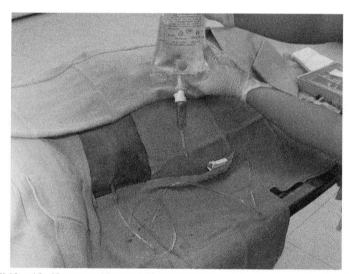

Fig. 6.24. Instill 10 to 15 ml/kg warmed Lactated Ringer's or 0.9% sodium chloride solution into the abdominal cavity. Watch carefully for signs of pain or respiratory distress. If able, walk the patient around for several minutes. If the patient is not ambulatory, then gently roll the patient from side to side to distribute the fluid evenly within the peritoneal cavity.

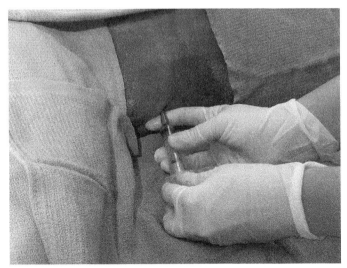

Fig. 6.25. Fluid can be aspirated from the abdomen with a routine four-quadrant abdominocentesis. Alternatively, if the catheter is going to be used for multiple lavages, for example, a patient with pancreatitis, the catheter can be secured to the body wall with a purse-string suture, then taped in place.

ABDOMINAL DRAINAGE CATHETER

Introduction

Placement of a temporary abdominal drainage catheter is useful in situations of temporary peritoneal dialysis or drainage of uroabdomen. The drainage catheter can be used until definitive exploratory laparotomy can be performed, or until the catheter becomes clogged with omentum.

Supplies Needed

Electric clippers and blades
Sterile field towels (4)
Backhaus towel clamps (4)
Number 10 scalpel blade
Scalpel handle
3-ml syringe with 3/4- to 1-1/2-inch needle (22-gauge)
2% lidocaine
Curved mosquito hemostats
Thumb forceps
Mayo scissors
Argyle trocarized thoracic drainage tube OR (16 to 22) Fr
Red rubber catheter (16 to 22 Fr)
2–0 nylon suture
3–0 absorbable suture
Christmas tree adapter
1-ml syringe
IV infusion tubing
Sterile bag for collection and drainage of fluid
Antimicrobial ointment

Indications

Temporary drainage of uroabdomen until definitive repair of urethral or urinary bladder leakage is performed
Intermittent lavage and dilution of inflammatory processes such as peritonitis

Contraindications

Known bowel perforation or septic peritonitis
Hypoalbuminemia

 Video available online

Go to www.wiley.com/go/hackett to view a video of this procedure.

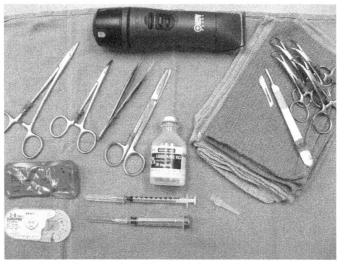

Fig. 6.26. Equipment needed for placement of an abdominal drainage catheter.

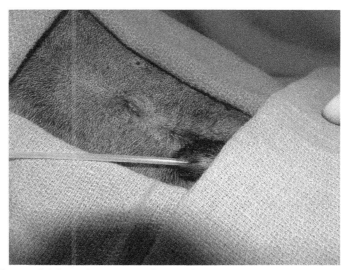

Fig. 6.27. Clip the ventral abdomen from the level of the umbilicus caudally to the level of the pubis and laterally to the folds of the flank. In male dogs, it is beneficial to place a urinary catheter first.

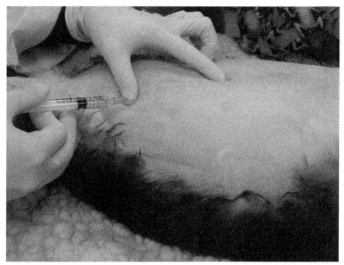

Fig. 6.28. Aseptically scrub the clipped area, then drape with sterile field towels secured with towel clamps. Infuse 1 mg/kg 2% lidocaine mixed with a trace of sodium bicarbonate just caudal and to the right of the umbilicus. Insert the needle through the ventral abdominal musculature and infuse the local anesthetic as you withdraw the needle.

Helpful hint: Disconnect the syringe from the needle so that you remember where your tunnel of local anesthetic has been infused.

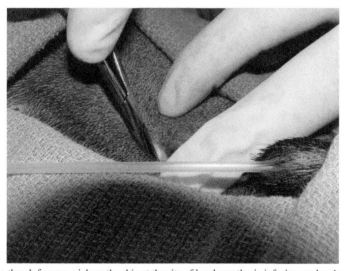

Fig. 6.29. With a thumb forceps, pick up the skin at the site of local anesthesia infusion, and make a stab incision through the skin into the subcutaneous tissue with a number 10 scalpel blade.

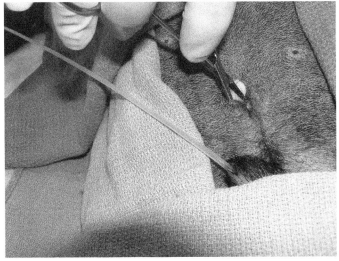

Fig. 6.30. Bluntly dissect through the subcutaneous tissue to the level of the external rectus abdominal muscles with mosquito hemostats.

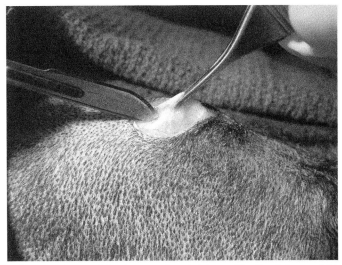

Fig. 6.31. Visualize the external rectus abdominus muscle and pick up with a thumb forceps. Make a small stab incision through the rectus abdominus with a number 10 scalpel blade into the peritoneal cavity.

(a)

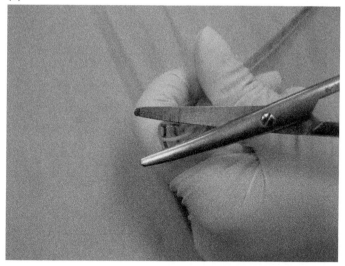

(b)

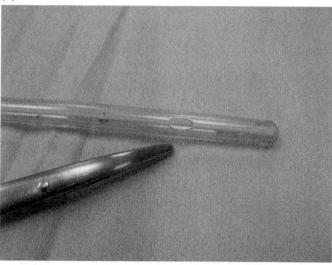

Figs. 6.32a–b. Cut additional side-holes in either an Argyle trocarized thoracic drain tube or a red rubber catheter, making sure that none of the holes is larger than 50% of the circumference of the catheter to prevent iatrogenic weakening.

Helpful hint: If an Argyle catheter is used, make sure that the most proximal hole is located on the radio-opaque stripe, so that you can make sure that the entire functional length of the tube is within the peritoneal cavity and to check if the tube has migrated.

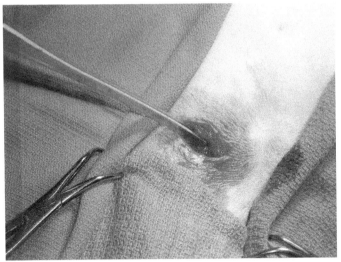

Fig. 6.33. Insert either an Argyle trocarized thoracic drainage catheter or a red rubber catheter into which additional side-ports have been cut into the peritoneal cavity.

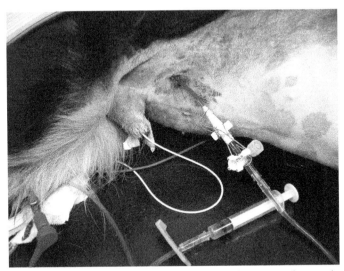

Fig. 6.34. Immediately connect the proximal end of the catheter to a Christmas tree adapter or 1-ml syringe casing connected to an IV infusion set and closed collection bag.

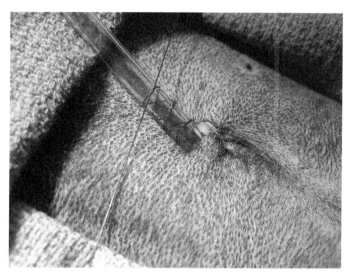

Fig. 6.35. Using absorbable suture, secure a purse-string suture into the external rectus abdominus around the tube. Make sure that the suture is not too tight to prevent tube removal at a later date. Using nonabsorbable suture, secure a second purse-string suture in the skin around the tube. Leave the ends of the suture long, and create a finger-trap suture around the tube.

> **Helpful hint:** Make sure that the throws of suture and knots pinch or crimp the tube snugly, to prevent tube migration.

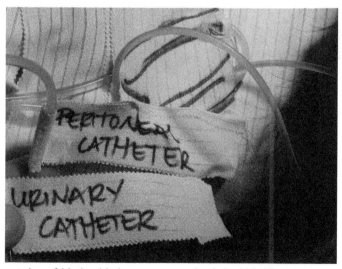

Fig. 6.36. Place a cut piece of 4-inch × 4-inch gauze square and antimicrobial ointment over the tube entrance site. Bandage the tube to the abdomen with layers of cotton roll gauze, Kling, and Elastikon®, or Vetrap™.

> **Helpful hint:** Make sure that the cranial layer of adhesive tape adheres to a piece of fur, to prevent the bandage from migrating caudally. Label the bandage and draw the outline of the tube to prevent iatrogenic cutting of the tube during bandage removal for bandage change.

REFERENCES

Connally HE. Cytology and fluid analysis of the acute abdomen. *Clin Tech Small Anim Pract* 18(1):39–44, 2003.

Crowe DT. Diagnostic abdominal paracentesis techniques: clinical evaluation in 129 dogs and cats. *J American Anim Hosp Assoc* 20:223–230, 1984.

Crowe DT. Abdominocentesis and diagnostic peritoneal lavage in small animals. *Modern Vet Pract* 13:877–882, 1984.

Walters JM. Abdominal paracentesis and diagnostic peritoneal lavage. *Clin Tech Small Anim Pract* 18(1):32–38, 2003.

CHAPTER 7

Pericardiocentesis and Pericardial Drainage Catheter

INTRODUCTION

Pericardial tamponade and the presence of even small amounts of fluid within the pericardial space can greatly impede cardiac preload and subsequently, cardiac output. The recognition of and rapid removal of pericardial effusion can be life-saving in some patients.

Supplies Needed

Electric clippers and blades
Antimicrobial scrub solution
3- or 6-ml syringe with 22-gauge, 3/4-inch needle
Number 11 scalpel blade
Abbott 16-gauge long over-the-needle catheter OR
Turkel drainage catheter
30- or 60-ml catheter-tip syringe
Three-way stop-cock
Intravenous extension tubing
Bowl or graduated cylinder for collection
Red-topped and EDTA tubes
ECG monitor
Optional supplies: Nonabsorbable suture on cutting needle

Indications

Pericardial effusion impairing cardiac preload and
cardiac output
Diagnosis of inflammatory and neoplastic effusions

Contraindications

Coagulopathies secondary to Vitamin K antagonist rodenticide intoxication

 Video available online

Go to www.wiley.com/go/hackett to view a video of this procedure.

Veterinary Emergency and Critical Care Procedures, Second Edition. Timothy B. Hackett and Elisa M. Mazzaferro.
© 2012 John Wiley & Sons, Inc. Published 2012 by John Wiley & Sons, Inc.

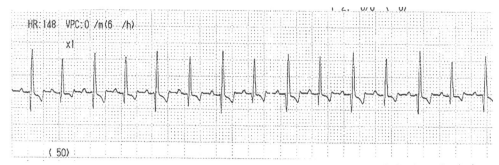

HR:148 VPC:0 /m(6 /h)
x1

(50)

Fig. 7.1. Electrical alternans is a characteristic ECG abnormality observed when the heart is floating and swinging within the fluid in the pericardial sac, creating small, then larger ECG complexes. Low-amplitude ECG waveforms can also be associated with pericardial effusion, although they are also associated with severe obesity, hypothyroidism, hypothermia, and hypovolemic shock.

(a)

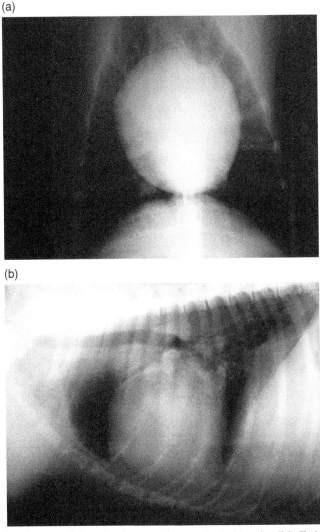

(b)

Figs. 7.2a–b. Ventrodorsal and lateral thoracic radiographs from a patient with pericardial effusion, demonstrating a large globoid cardiac silhouette.

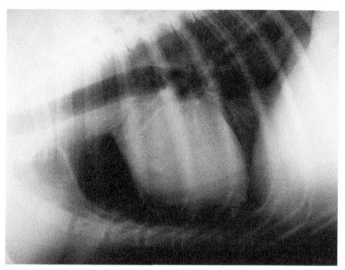

Fig. 7.3. Lateral thoracic radiograph from a dog with minimal pericardial effusion. Note the relatively normal cardiac silhouette, and the enlarged caudal vena cava.

Helpful hint: The cardiac silhouette may appear normal in the ventrodorsal, dorsoventral, or lateral radiographs if pericardial effusion is acute, leading to severe cardiovascular compromise without radiographic appearance of abnormalities. In such cases, the enlarged caudal vena cava on thoracic radiographs may be the only clue that pericardial effusion is present.

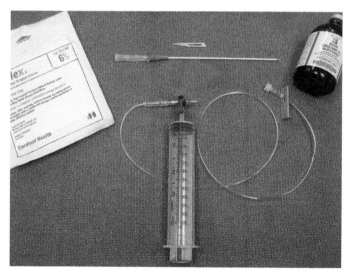

Fig. 7.4. Supplies needed to perform a pericardiocentesis include a number 11 scalpel blade; 2% lidocaine; 3- or 6-ml syringe; 22-gauge, 3/4- inch needle; electric clippers and blades; antimicrobial scrub solution; a Abbott large-bore (14 or 16 gauge) over-the needle catheter; ECG; three-way stop-cock; IV extension tubing; 30- or 60-ml syringe; and red- and lavender-topped tubes. Whenever possible, perform a prothrombin time prior to performing any pericardiocentesis, because vitamin K antagonist rodenticide intoxication can cause hemorrhagic pericardial effusion.

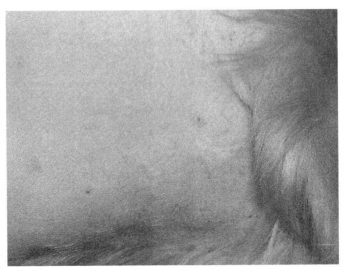

Fig. 7.5. Clip a large area of fur caudal to the elbow on the right lateral thoracic wall, over the fifth to eighth ribs.

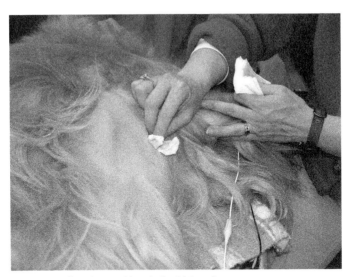

Fig. 7.6. Aseptically scrub the clipped area with antimicrobial scrub.

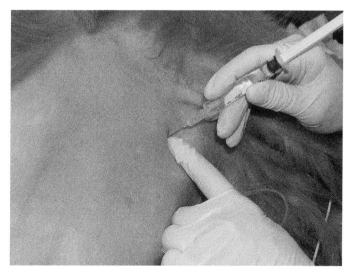

Fig. 7.7. Insert a bleb of lidocaine dorsal to the sternum and just caudal to the point of the elbow or at the sixth intercostal space.

Helpful hint: Make sure that you infuse the local anesthetic into the intercostal muscles and infuse as you draw the needle out, creating a tunnel of anesthetized tissue through which to insert your needle.

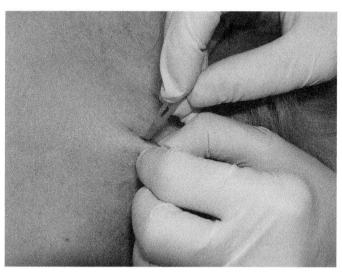

Fig. 7.8. Rescrub the clipped area and drape with field towels secured with towel clamps. Make a small stab incision through the skin where you infused the local anesthetic.

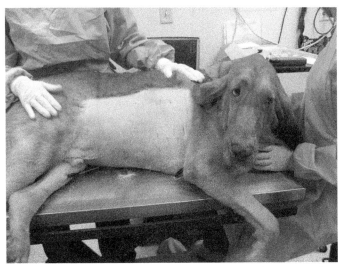

Fig. 7.9. Attach the patient to an ECG monitor, if available, to monitor for cardiac dysrhythmias while performing the pericardiocentesis.

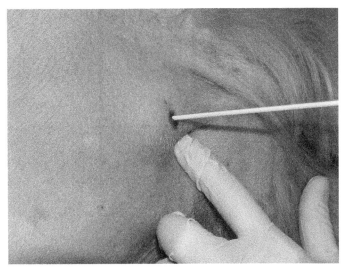

Fig. 7.10. Insert the over-the-needle catheter through the skin incision and through the body wall in the anesthetized area of muscle. Watch carefully for dysrhythmias on the ECG monitor, and for a flash of blood in the hub of the needle.

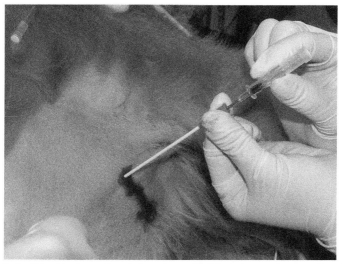

Fig. 7.11. Once a flash of blood is observed, push the catheter off of the stylette, and remove the stylette. Attach the hub of the catheter to the length of IV extension tubing, and draw the fluid off the pericardial sac.

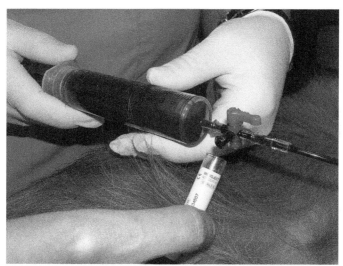

Fig. 7.12. Place a small amount of the pericardial fluid in the red- and lavender-topped tubes for fluids analysis. Watch the red-topped tube carefully for the presence of a clot. Clot formation may indicate an active bleed, but more commonly, suggests that you have inserted the catheter into the heart itself, and not the pericardium. Set aside some of the fluid for culture, in the event that the fluid is due to an infectious cause.

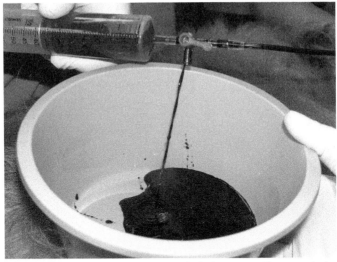

Fig. 7.13. Removal of even a small amount of blood can drastically improve cardiac output by improving cardiac filling.

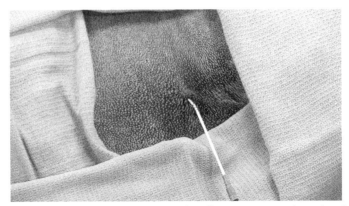

Fig. 7.14. The pericardial catheter can be sutured in place with a finger trap suture, to intermittently drain pericardial effusion in a patient that is actively bleeding.

REFERENCES

Beardow AW. The diagnostic and therapeutic approach to the patient with acute congestive heart failure. *Clin Tech Small Anim Pract* 15(2):70–75, 2000.

Bouvy BM, Bjorling DE. Pericardial effusion in dogs and cats: Part II. *Comp Contin Educ Pract Vet* 13(4):633–642, 1991.

Gidlewski J, Petrie JP. Pericardiocentesis and principles of echocardiographic imaging in the patient with cardiac neoplasia. *Clin Tech Sm Anim Pract* 18(2):131–134, 2003.

Johnson S, Martin M, Binns S, Day MJ. A retrospective study of clinical findings, treatment, and outcome in 143 dogs with pericardial effusion. *J Sm Anim Pract* 45(11):546–552, 2004.

Macintire DK, Drobatz KJ, Haskins SC, Saxon WD. Chapter 10, Cardiac emergencies. In: *Manual of Small Animal Emergency and Critical Care Medicine*. Philadelphia: Lippincott, Williams, and Wilkins. pp. 161–162, 2005.

CHAPTER 8

Central Venous Pressure

INTRODUCTION

In the absence of vascular obstruction, central venous pressure (CVP) is the measure of the hydrostatic pressure within the thoracic vena cava. Central venous pressure often is used as an indicator of vascular preload, or the volume of blood/fluid within the vascular space. Central venous pressure also is affected by the contractile function of the right heart, the change in intrathoracic pressure throughout the phases of respiration, positive pressure ventilation, upper airway obstruction, and the cardiac cycle.

Because pulmonary artery catheters are not routinely used in veterinary medicine, people often use changes in a patient's CVP as a rough indicator or reflection of the potential for pulmonary vascular overload. It is to be noted, however, that CVP is a measure of right heart function, and does not directly measure left heart function at all. Normal CVP is 0 to 5 cm H_2O. Values less than 0 cm H_2O reflect hypovolemia or peripheral vasodilation, and values greater than 16 cm H_2O are associated with right-sided cardiac failure. The CVP measurement should be used to monitor trends in intravascular volume and right-sided cardiac function and used to gauge fluid resuscitation. As a rule, a patient's CVP should not increase by more than 5 cm H_2O during any 24-hour period to avoid pulmonary vascular overload. If a central venous catheter cannot be placed in a patient's jugular vein, a long catheter in the medial saphenous vein in cats and small dogs can be used to monitor trends in CVP.

Supplies Needed

Electric clippers
Electric clipper blades
Antimicrobial scrub
4- × 4-inch gauze squares
Central venous catheter

Veterinary Emergency and Critical Care Procedures, Second Edition. Timothy B. Hackett and Elisa M. Mazzaferro.
© 2012 John Wiley & Sons, Inc. Published 2012 by John Wiley & Sons, Inc.

Cotton roll gauze
Kling or gauze bandage material
Elastikon® or Vetrap™
T-port
IV extension tubing (2)
Heparinized 0.9% saline flush
20-ml syringe
3-way stopcock
Manometer or ruler

Indications

Monitor fluid therapy in cases of:
  Septic shock
  Cardiac disease
  Renal failure
  Severe hypovolemia

Contraindications

Coagulopathies
  Thrombocytopenia
  Thromobocytopathia
  Vitamin K antagonist rodenticide intoxication
Hypercoagulable states
  Hyperadrenocorticism
  Protein-losing nephropathy
  Protein-losing enteropathy
  Immune-mediated hemolytic anemia
Elevated intracranial pressure
  Head trauma
  Intracranial mass lesions
  Intractable seizures

 Video available online

Go to www.wiley.com/go/hackett to view a video of this procedure.

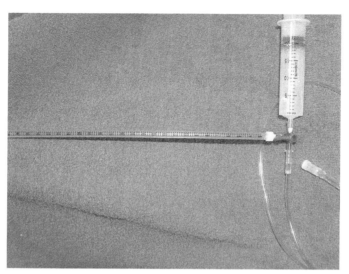

Fig. 8.1. Supplies needed for central catheter and central venous pressure (CVP) measurement.

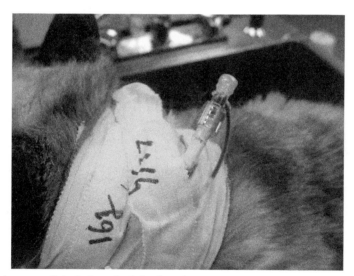

Fig. 8.2. Central venous catheter in the patient's jugular vein.

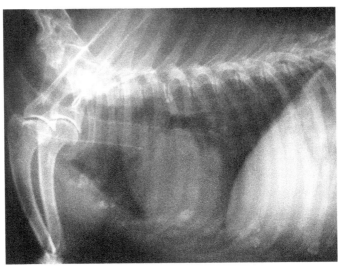

Fig. 8.3. Lateral thoracic radiograph confirming correct placement of a jugular catheter for CVP measurements. For accurate CVP measurements, the tip of the jugular catheter should lie just outside of the right atrium of the heart.

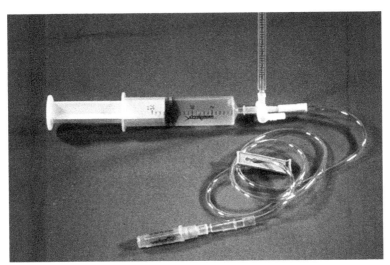

Fig. 8.4. Connect the female end of a length of IV extension tubing to the male port of a three-way stopcock. Connect either a flushed length of IV extension tubing OR a manometer to one of the female ports of the three-way stopcock. Connect a 20-ml syringe of heparinized 0.9% saline to the other female port of the three-way stopcock.

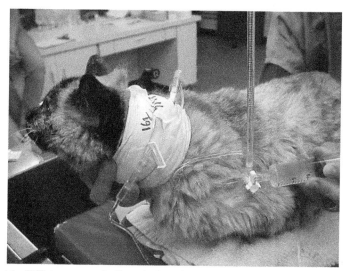

Fig. 8.5. Connect the CVP apparatus to the T-port in the patient's jugular catheter.

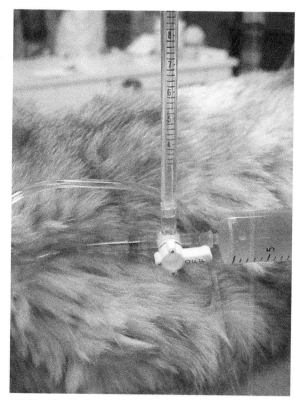

Fig. 8.6. Lower the 0 cm H_2O mark to the level of the patient's manubrium when the patient is in lateral recumbency, and at the point of the elbow for a patient in sternal recumbency. Whatever method you use, make sure that the same method and patient positioning is used for all subsequent measurements.

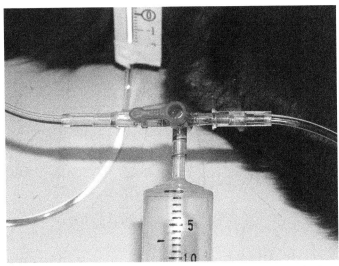

Fig. 8.7. Turn the stopcock OFF to the manometer, and ON to the patient, to flush the patient's catheter with a small amount of heparinized saline.

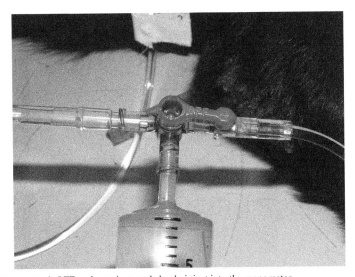

Fig. 8.8. Turn the stopcock OFF to the patient, and slowly inject into the manometer.

Helpful hint: Use care to not create any air bubbles that will interfere with accurate CVP measurement.

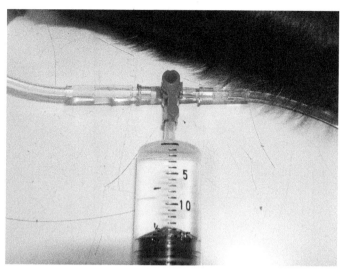

Fig. 8.9. Again, lower the 0 cm H$_2$O point on the manometer to the level of the patient's manubrium (or shoulder, if in sternal recumbency), and turn the stopcock OFF to the syringe. The fluid column in the manometer will equilibrate with the column of fluid in the patient's vascular space.

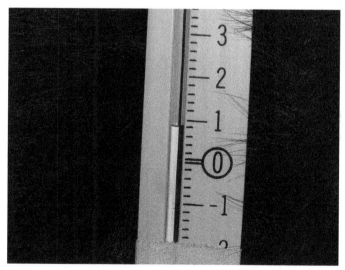

Fig. 8.10. Once the column of fluid in the manometer stops decreasing and rises and falls with the patient's heartbeat, measure the level on the lower point of the meniscus in the manometer to obtain the CVP measurement. Repeat the process three to five times to confirm the accuracy of the measurement, because outliers can occur.

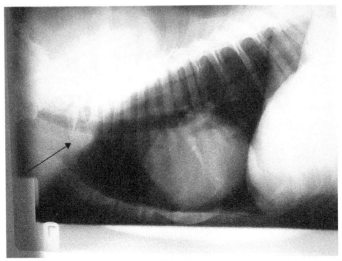

Fig. 8.11. The tip of this jugular catheter is not just outside of the right atrium. Thus, it is not ideal for measurement of central venous pressure. Similarly, catheters that are inserted too far into the heart are not ideal for measurement of central venous pressure.

REFERENCES

Jennings PB, Anderson RW, Martin AM. Central venous pressure monitoring: a guide to blood volume replacement in the dog. *J Am Vet Med Assoc* 151:1283–1293, 1967.

Machon RG, Raffee MR, Robinson EP. Central venous pressure measurements in the caudal vena cava of sedated cats. *J Vet Emerg Crit Care* 5(2):121–129, 1995.

Oakley RE, Olivier B, Eyster GE, et al. Experimental evaluation of central venous pressure monitoring in the dog. *J Am Anim Hosp Assoc* 33:77–82, 1997.

Waddell LS. Direct blood pressure monitoring. *Clin Tech Sm Anim Pract* 15(3):111–118, 2000.

CHAPTER 9

Cardiopulmonary Resuscitation

INTRODUCTION

Cardiopulmonary resuscitation (CPR) can make the difference between life and death in a dying animal. Cardiopulmonary resuscitation involves administration of supplemental oxygen and artificial ventilation and manual thoracic or cardiac compressions to deliver oxygen from the lungs to the peripheral tissues (namely, the brain and the heart) during cessation of spontaneous and effective respiration and cardiac output. In addition, by providing circulation, carbon dioxide and other waste products from the peripheral tissues are delivered to the lungs and into the external environment. Depending on the cause of respiratory and cardiac arrest, operators have a 3% to 28% chance of success, provided that the condition that has caused the respiratory and/or cardiac arrest can be immediately reversed.

Supplies Needed

3- to 12-ml syringes
22-gauge hypodermic needles
ECG
Capnograph
Various sized endotracheal tubes
Gauze to secure endotracheal tube
Laryngoscope
Drugs
    Atropine
    Epinephrine
    Naloxone
    Yohimbine or atipamezole
    Sodium bicarbonate

Veterinary Emergency and Critical Care Procedures, Second Edition. Timothy B. Hackett and Elisa M. Mazzaferro.
© 2012 John Wiley & Sons, Inc. Published 2012 by John Wiley & Sons, Inc.

Indications

Loss of spontaneous ventilation and cardiac output

Contraindications

Irreversible underlying process has caused the cardiopulmonary arrest
   End-stage cancer
   End-stage renal or hepatic disease
   End-stage neurologic disease
   End-stage cardiac or pulmonary disease
   Sepsis or systemic inflammatory response syndrome (SIRS)
   Disseminated intravascular coagulation (DIC)
   Acute respiratory distress syndrome (ARDS)

CLOSED-CHEST CPR

(1) Place the patient in lateral or dorsal recumbency. The position is largely dependent on the patient size (dorsal recumbency for patients < 15 kg, lateral recumbency for patients > 15 kg) and the shape of the thorax. For example, deep-chested breeds, even those patients < 15 kg, may do better in lateral recumbency, or in a V-trough, to prevent side-to-side movement during external thoracic compression.

(2) Have an assistant palpate for a femoral arterial pulse. If no pulse is palpable during thoracic compression, the position should be changed and the strength of compression should be increased.

(3) Using a laryngoscope, intubate the patient and tie the endotracheal tube in place. Inflate the cuff of the endotracheal tube, and attach to an oxygen source.

> **Helpful hint:** One of the most common mistakes made during CPR is failure to use a laryngoscope to intubate the patient, which results in esophageal intubation.

(4) Breathe for the patient 15 to 20 times per minute.

(5) Insert a 22- or 25-gauge needle through the nasal philtrum to the level of the periosteum and twist. This acupressure point has also been called "Gen Chung," and is used to help stimulate spontaneous respiration.

(6) If available, attach the endotracheal tube to a capnograph to visualize the success of perfusion.

(7) Hook up an ECG monitor to the patient and moisten with gel.

> **Helpful hint:** If an electrical defibrillator is available, use care to avoid isopropyl alcohol on the ECG leads, because flames can result during defibrillation.

(8)   Have an assistant to draw up drugs as necessary using the following guide:

Atropine:	0.04 mg/kg IV, IT, IO
Epinephrine:	0.02 to 0.04 mg/kg IV, IT, IO
Naloxone:	0.01 to 0.04 mg/kg IV, IT, IO
Atipamezole:	0.05 mg/kg IV, IT, IO
Yohimbine:	0.11 mg/kg IV
Sodium bicarbonate:	1 mEq/kg IV or IO, NOT IT

> **Helpful hint:** All of the above drugs EXCEPT for sodium bicarbonate can be administered into the trachea if vascular access is not available.

> **Helpful hint:** Have a crash cart or box stocked with needles, syringes, and all of the drugs necessary for easy access and use in CPR. Also, have a number of endotracheal tubes of various sizes, along with a laryngoscope, available for easy access. A book with drug doses in milligrams and milliliters is invaluable during a cardiopulmonary arrest.

(9)   To administer drugs into the trachea, insert a rigid polypropylene catheter into the endotracheal tube to the level of the patient's carina, and instill the drug, followed by 5 ml to 10 ml of sterile 0.9% saline. Next, breathe into the endotracheal tube with an ambu-bag, anesthetic circuit, or an assistant's breath.

(10) If no return of spontaneous circulation occurs within two to three minutes of initiating CPR, the decision must be made whether to perform open chest CPR.

> **Helpful hint:** In the following circumstances, open-chest CPR should be initiated immediately:
>
> Obesity
> Pneumothorax
> Pericardial effusion
> Penetrating thoracic wound
> Hemothorax
> Flail chest
> Rib fractures
> Diaphragmatic hernia
> Unwitnessed cardiac arrest

> **Helpful hint:** If the underlying process that has caused cardiopulmonary arrest cannot be reversed almost immediately (electrolyte or acid-base disturbances, trauma, vasovagal event, anesthetic-related arrest, hypovolemia), the likelihood of being successful with closed- or open-chest CPR is less than 2%.

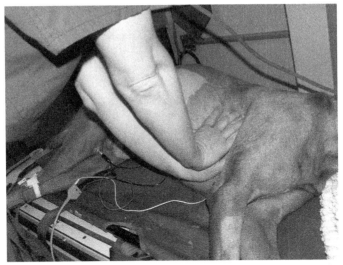

Fig. 9.1. Place one hand over the other and clasp the to – 120 times per minute. Compress the thorax approximately 30% of its diameter.

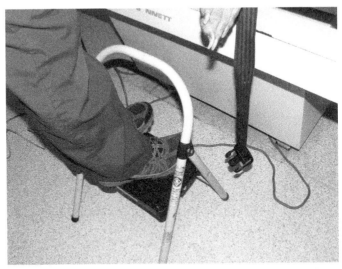

Fig. 9.2a. Stand on a stool or kneel on a table to get more leverage when performing thoracic compressions.

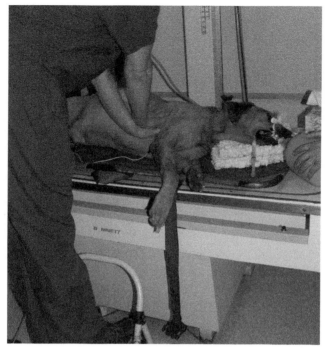

Fig. 9.2b. Remember to lock the elbows and push with the weight of the torso, rather than bending the elbows and using the strength of the forearms alone, to compress the thorax.

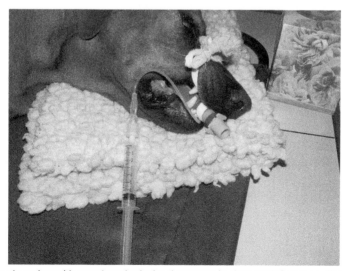

Fig. 9.3. Intubate the patient with an endotracheal tube, then secure in place and inflate the cuff to allow for positive pressure manual ventilation.

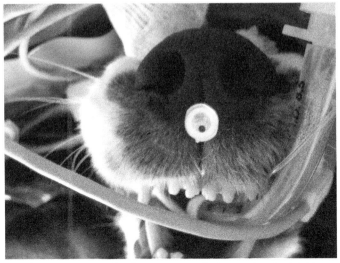

Fig. 9.4. "Gen Chung" is an acupressure point. Spontaneous respiration may be stimulated in some patients by placing a needle through the nasal philtrum to the level of the periosteum of the rostral maxilla and intermittently twisting.

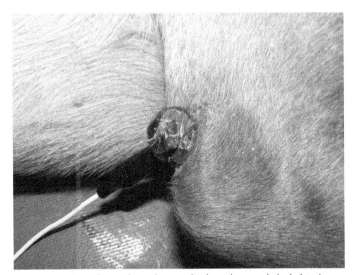

Fig. 9.5. Secure ECG leads on the patient and use ultrasound gel, not isopropyl alcohol, to improve contact with the skin. Isopropyl alcohol is flammable, and can cause iatrogenic burning of skin and fur during electrical defibrillation.

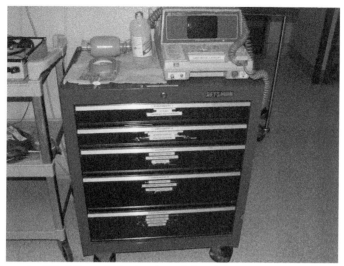

Fig. 9.6. A crash cart should be fully stocked and ready at all times in the event of an emergency.

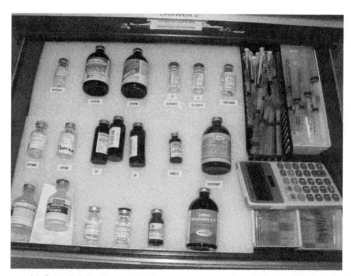

Fig. 9.7a. A drawer with foam that has been cut to have secure spaces for all drugs minimizes the inefficiency of searching for a particular item during CPR.

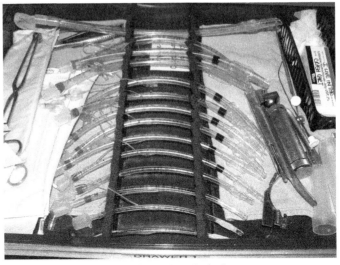

Fig. 9.7b. Drawer of a crash cart stocked with various endotracheal tubes.

Helpful hint: Make sure that the cuffs of all tubes are intact and functional.

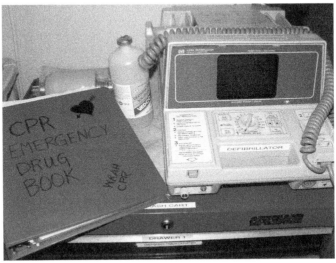

Fig. 9.8. A book of drugs, with dose charts for various size animals, is helpful in CPR. Give drug doses in both milliliters and milligrams for ease of drawing up in an emergency.

OPEN-CHEST CPR

Supplies

Electric clipper and blades
Number 10 scalpel blade
Mayo scissors
Finechetto retractors
Rumel tourniquet
Red rubber catheter (3 or 5–1/2 French)
Hemostat forceps
Absorbable suture (varying sizes)
Nonabsorbable suture or surgical staples
0.9% sterile saline
Suction apparatus

(1) Place the patient in right lateral recumbency.
(2) Clip, then scrub one clipper blade width at the point of the elbow on the left lateral thoracic wall. This will help prevent the scalpel blade from dulling.

> **Helpful hint:** Rather than count rib spaces to the fifth to seventh intercostal space, simply pull the elbow back to where it bends. This is the fifth to seventh intercostal space. This technique can help save valuable time.

(3) Make an incision through the skin and underlying fascia and muscle, starting dorsally to ventrally over the fifth to seventh intercostal space.
(4) Ask your assistant to stop breathing for the patient, and make a stab incision through the intercostal muscles into the pleural space with the tips of a Mayo scissors.
(5) Using the tips of the Mayo scissors in a sliding motion, extend the intercostal incision dorsally and ventrally.
(6) Clip the ribs at the cartilaginous portion of the costochondral junction and push the ribs under the adjacent ribs to improve visualization and enhance access to the heart.

> **Helpful hint:** Finechetto rib spreader retractors can also be used to open the intercostal space.

(7) Visualize the phrenic nerve as it passes over the heart.

> **Helpful hint:** Avoid the phrenic nerve, because damage to it will decrease the chance of spontaneous respiration.

(8) Pick up the pericardium at the apex of the heart, and using the Mayo scissors, make a small incision in the pericardial sac.
(9) Push your fingers into the incision made in the pericardium, and rip the pericardium away from the heart.
(10) Grasp the heart in your hand as if you are shaking someone's hand.

> **Helpful hint:** Use caution to avoid pulling the heart away from the great vessels.

(11)   Squeeze the heart from apex to base as it fills.
(12)   Watch for return of spontaneous circulation both by looking directly at the heart as well as the ECG monitor.
(13)   The descending aorta can be cross-clamped by placing a Rumel tourniquet or red rubber catheter around it. The tourniquet or catheter should be released to allow circulation to the caudal half of the body every seven minutes.

> **Helpful hint:** If a Rumel tourniquet or red rubber catheter is not available, your wrist can be used to compress the descending aorta while simultaneously compressing the heart.

> **Helpful hint:** Even with the heart directly in your hand, intracardiac injections should never be attempted inadvertent administration of any drug into the epicardium or myocardium can result in a more irritable focus of electrical activity, and worsen the change of return to spontaneous circulation.

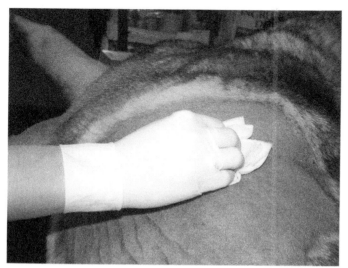

Fig. 9.9. Place the patient in right lateral recumbency and clip the fur on the lateral thorax caudal to the elbow.

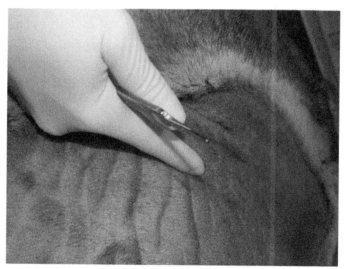

Fig. 9.10. Palpate the point of the elbow, at the fifth to seventh intercostal space.

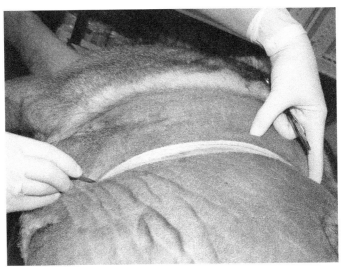

Fig. 9.11. Using a number 10 scalpel blade, make an incision through the skin and underlying subcutaneous tissue and intercostal muscles at the fifth to seventh intercostal space.

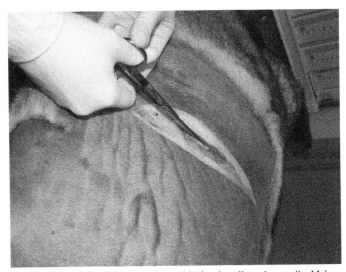

Fig. 9.12. Insert a Mayo scissors into the pleural cavity, and incise dorsally and ventrally. Make sure that the person who is performing manual ventilation stops breathing while you insert the Mayo scissors into the pleural space to avoid iatrogenic lung laceration.

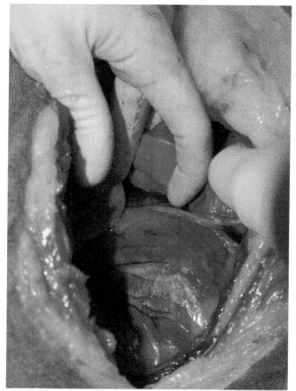

Fig. 9.13. Visualize the heart and lungs in the pleural cavity. The phrenic nerve can be visualized at the dorsal aspect of the heart.

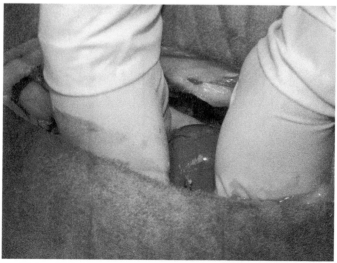

Fig. 9.14. After incising the pericardial sac, grasp the heart in both hands, if possible, and squeeze from apex to base.

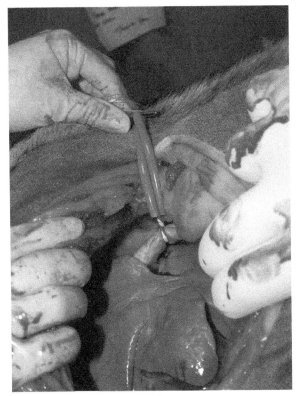

Fig. 9.15. A Rumel tourniquet can be used to occlude the descending aorta.

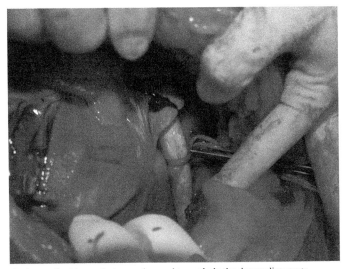

Fig. 9.16. Alternatively, a red rubber catheter can be used to occlude the descending aorta.

CLOSING THE THORAX IF RETURN OF SPONTANEOUS CIRCULATION OCCURS AFTER OPEN-CHEST CPR

(1) Lavage the thorax with copious amounts of 0.9% sterile saline solution warmed to body temperature.

(2) The pericardial sac can be left open.

(3) Place a red rubber or Argyle thoracic drainage catheter in the thorax, with the tube entrance caudal to the intercostal incision.

(4) Taking the blunt end of a swaged-on needle, push the needle through the intercostal space adjacent to the rib and around the adjacent rib. Pull the suture together and hold with a hemostat forceps.

(5) Repeat step 3 multiple times, closing the ribs and intercostal incision.

(6) Once all of the sutures and hemostats are in place, individually ligate each suture.

(7) Next, close the fascia above the intercostal space in a continuous layer with absorbable suture.

(8) Continue closing the underlying tissue in multiple layers of absorbable suture in a continuous pattern. The number of layers depends on how much underlying tissue is present.

(9) Close the subcutaneous tissue as directed above.

(10) Close the subcuticular tissue in a continuous pattern using absorbable suture (3–0).

(11) Close the skin with skin staples or Ford-interlocking nonabsorbable suture.

(12) Evacuate the thorax of any residual air, and keep thoracic drain in place for a minimum of 12 hours or overnight. Intermittently aspirate the tube to ensure no residual pneumothorax is present.

(a)

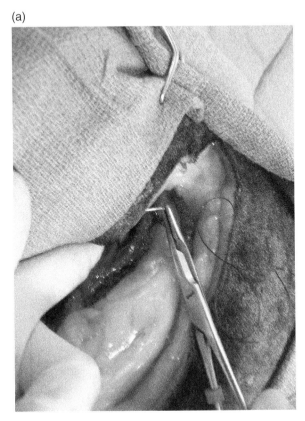

(b)

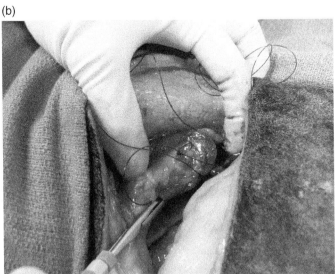

Figs. 9.17a–b. Take the blunt end of the swaged-on needle and pass it through the intercostal muscle and tissue, around the rib, and again through the intercostal tissue of the rib adjacent to it.

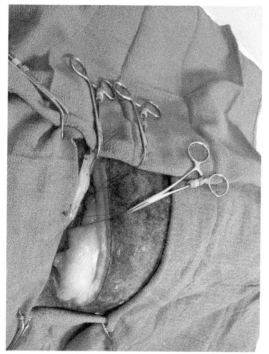

Fig. 9.18. Secure the suture with hemostat forceps, and repeat several times.

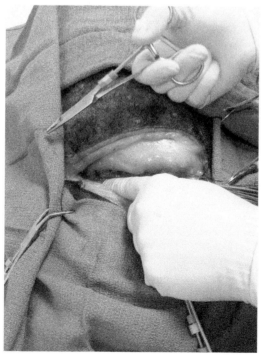

Fig. 9.19. Secure the sutures, one at a time, to close the intercostal muscles.

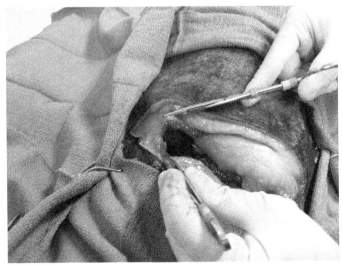

Fig. 9.20. Suture the subcutaneous tissue with absorbable suture in a continuous pattern.

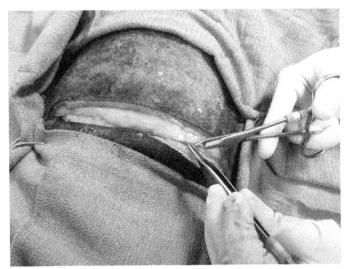

Fig. 9.21. Continue to close the subcutaneous tissue in layers, using absorbable suture in a continuous pattern.

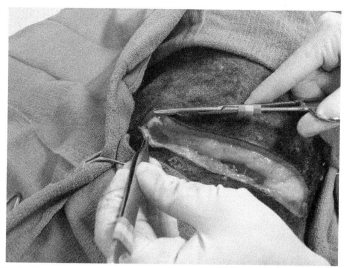
Fig. 9.22. Close the final subcutaneous layer as previously described.

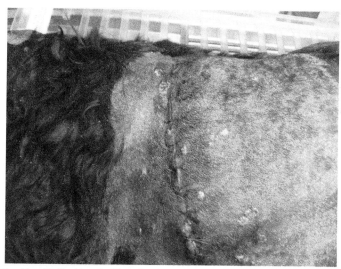
Fig. 9.23. Close the skin with Ford interlocking, simple continuous sutures or surgical staples.

REFERENCES

Boller M, Boller EM, Oodegard S, Otto CM. Small animal cardiopulmonary resuscitation requires a continuum of care: proposal for a chain of survival for veterinary students. *J Am Vet Med Assoc* 240(5):540–554, 2012.

Boller M. Celebrating the 50th anniversary of cardiopulmonary resuscitation: from animals to humans.... and back? *J Vet Emerg Crit Care* 20:553–557, 2010.

Cole SG, Otto CM, Hughes D. Cardiopulmonary cerebral resuscitation in small animals–a clinical practice review. Part I. *J Vet Emerg Crit Care* 12:261–267, 2002.

Cole SG, Otto CM, Hughes D. Cardiopulmonary cerebral resuscitation in small animals–a clinical practice review. Part II. *J Vet Emerg Crit Care* 13:13–23, 2003.

Hofmeister EH, Brainard BM, Egger CM, et al. Prognostic indicators for dogs and cats with cardiopulmonary arrest treated by cadiopulmonary cerebral resuscitation at a university teaching hospital. *J Am Vet Med Assoc* 235:50–57, 2009.

Waldrop JE, Rozanski EA, Swanke ED, et al. Causes of cardiopulmonary arrest, resuscitation management, and functional outcome in dogs and cats surviving cardiopulmonary arrest. *J Vet Emerg Crit Care* 14:22–29, 2004.

CHAPTER 10

Continuous Rate Infusions

INTRODUCTION

For some drugs, it is necessary to maintain constant plasma and tissue levels and pharmacologic effect. Infusions minimize fluctuations in drug levels. Drugs with a narrow therapeutic spectrum, and those with rapid onset and elimination, can be titrated to the individual patient with continuous intravenous administration. Continuous rate infusions (CRI) can be administered using an intravenous drip set or infusion pump system.

Drugs are given at continuous rate infusions for sedation, analgesia, anesthesia, pressor and inotropic support, and antiarrhythmic therapy (Table 10.1). For simplicity, drugs can be mixed into the patients' daily maintenance fluids. Careful attention to units is necessary to ensure accuracy when formulating infusions.

PHARMACOKINETICS

Drug levels in plasma begin to rise when an intravenous continuous rate infusion begins. A plateau of plasma drug concentration is reached when the rate of administration matches the rate of elimination. This is known as steady state. A drug reaches steady state between five and seven elimination half-lives, with five corresponding to 95% of the steady state drug concentration and seven corresponding to 99% of the steady state drug concentration. The onset of drug action tends to occur at 3–1/3 half-lives, a time that corresponds to 90% of the steady state drug concentration.

Veterinary Emergency and Critical Care Procedures, Second Edition. Timothy B. Hackett and Elisa M. Mazzaferro.
© 2012 John Wiley & Sons, Inc. Published 2012 by John Wiley & Sons, Inc.

Table 10.1. Drugs commonly delivered by continuous rate infusion in veterinary medicine.

Drug	CRI dosage (µg/kg/min unless*, then U/kg/min)	Elimination half-life (hours)	Time to steady state 7 half-lives (hours)
Buprenorphine	0.017–0.05	5.9	41.3
Butorphanol	1.7–16.7	1.53	10.71
Diazepam	1.7–16.7	0.25	1.75
Diltiazem	5–20	5	35
Dobutamine	2–20	0.04	0.29
Dopamine	1–20	0.11	0.82
Fentanyl	0.05–0.3	2.6	18.3
Furosemide	2–15	1	7
Hydromorphone	0.17–0.83	0.57	3.99
Insulin (regular)	0.0015*	0.28	1.98
Isoproterenol	0.04–0.08	0.05	0.35
Ketamine	0.83–33.3	1.02	7.15
Lidocaine	15–80	1.73	12.13
Metoclopramide	0.04–0.3	1.5	10.5
Morphine	0.83–16.7	0.6	4.2
Norepinephrine	0.05–2	0.004	0.03
Procainamide	20–40	2.43	17
Propofol	50–400	1.33	9.33
Sodium nitroprusside	1–3	72	504
Vasopressin	0.0005–0.004*	0.09	0.63

CALCULATIONS

µg/kg/min infusions are converted to ml/hr pump rates using the following formulas:

$$\mu g/kg/min \times Body\ Wt\ (kg) = \mu g/min \times 60\ min/hr = \mu g/hr \div \mu g/ml\ of\ solution = ml/hr$$

To incorporate infusion into ml/hr total fluid requirements:

$$\mu g/kg/min \times Body\ Wt\ (kg) = \mu g/min \times 60\ min/hr = \mu g$$

added to known volume of crystalloid fluid administered by pump each hour

To convert concentration per volume to an equivalent drug dose in a larger dilution volume:

$$Volume\ solution_1\ (ml) \times Concentration_1\ (mg/ml) = Volume_2\ (ml) \times Concentration_2\ (mg/ml)$$

Web-based, smart phone, PDA, computer pad, or dedicated computer software CRI calculators can be used to minimize errors in drug calculation of commonly used infusions.

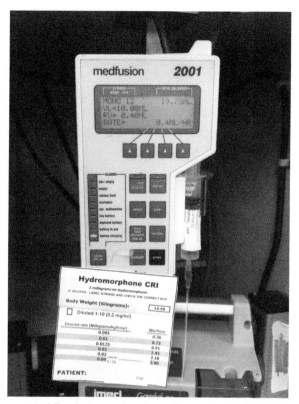

Fig. 10.1. A syringe pump set to deliver hydromorphone by continuous rate infusion. A spreadsheet-based drug calculator was used and a printout kept close to the patient. By using a syringe pump in line with the patient's maintenance fluids, the rate and amount of drug delivered can be adjusted without changing the fluid plan.

REFERENCES

Hackett TB, Hackett E. Constant rate infusions. In: Feldman EC (Ed): *Ettinger and Feldman's Textbook of Veterinary Internal Medicine* 7th *Edition*. St. Louis, MO: Elsevier. pp. 361–363, 2010.
Rowland M, Tozer TN. Continuous rate infusions. *Clinical Pharmacokinetics; Concepts and Applications 3rd Edition*. Philadelphia: Lippincott Williams and Wilkins. pp. 322–329, 1995.

Index

abdominal drainage catheter, 225–32
abdominocentesis, 209–13
airway pressure therapy, 157–60
antepubic cystostomy catheter, 171, 200–207
arterial catheter, 58–66
auricular arterial catheter, 64–6
auricular catheter, 35–8

Braun esophagostomy tube insertion
  device, 83

cardiopulmonary resuscitation, 253–72
central venous catheter, 1–20
central venous pressure, 243–51
cephalic venous catheter, 30–34
continuous rate infusion, 273–6
CPR, closed-chest, 254–60
CPR, open-chest, 261–6
CPR, thoracic wall closure, 267–71
CRI, 273–6
CRI calculation, 274
CVP, 243–51
cystostomy, 171, 200–207

diagnostic peritoneal lavage, 209, 214–24
diagnostic peritoneal lavage, over-the-wire,
  218–24

dorsal pedal arterial catheterization, 58–63
DPL, 209, 214–24
drug steady state, 273

electrical alternans, 234
esophagostomy tube, 75–86
EZ IO, 45, 53–7

flail chest, 101

Gen Chung, 258

intraosseous catheter, 45–57
intratracheal oxygen catheter, 144–8

jejunostomy tube, 91–5
jugular catheter, 3–9
J-wire, 25

lateral saphenous catheter, 9–14

manometer, 244–6
medial saphenous catheter, 15–20

nasal oxygen catheter, 133–9
nasoesophageal feeding tube, 69–74
nasogastric feeding tube, 69–74

Veterinary Emergency and Critical Care Procedures, Second Edition. Timothy B. Hackett and Elisa M. Mazzaferro.
© 2012 John Wiley & Sons, Inc. Published 2012 by John Wiley & Sons, Inc.

nasopharyngeal oxygen catheter,
  133–9
nutritional support, 69–86

open sucking chest wound, 122–5
orogastric lavage, 87–90
over-the-wire catheter, 21
oxygen hood, 140–143
oxygen supplementation, 133–48

parenteral nutrition, 96–8
PEEP, 157, 158, 160
percutaneous facilitation, 31
pericardial drainage catheter,
  233–41
pericardial effusion, 233–41
pericardial tamponade, 233–4
pericardiocentesis, 233–41
peripheral venous catheter, 29–38
pneumothorax, 101, 108
pneumothorax, tension, 101, 108
pressure volume curve, 158

rib fractures, local anesthesia, 126–31

Seldinger technique, 21–8

tension pneumothorax, 101, 108
thoracic drainage catheter, 108–22
thoracocentesis, 101–7
thoracostomy tube, 101, 108–21
tracheal oxygen catheter, 144–8
tracheostomy tube, 149–56
transoral wash, 161–4
transthoracic aspirate, 165–9

urinary catheter, 171–93
urinary catheter, female cat, 184, 191–3
urinary catheter, female dog, 177–83
urinary catheter, male cat, 184–90
urinary catheter, male dog, 173–6
urohydropulsion, 171, 194–9

vascular access techniques, 1–67
vascular cutdown, 39–44